T0210800

SpringerBriefs in Statistics

JSS Research Series in Statistics

The current research of statistics in Japan has expanded in several directions in line with recent trends in academic activities in the area of statistics and statistical sciences over the globe. The core of these research activities in statistics in Japan has been the Japan Statistical Society (JSS). This society, the oldest and largest academic organization for statistics in Japan, was founded in 1931 by a handful of pioneer statisticians and economists and now has a history of about 80 years. Many distinguished scholars have been members, including the influential statistician Hirotugu Akaike, who was a past president of JSS, and the notable mathematician Kiyosi Itô, who was an earlier member of the Institute of Statistical Mathematics (ISM), which has been a closely related organization since the establishment of ISM. The society has two academic journals: the Journal of the Japan Statistical Society (English Series) and the Journal of the Japan Statistical Society (Japanese Series). The membership of JSS consists of researchers, teachers, and professional statisticians in many different fields including mathematics, statistics, engineering, medical sciences, government statistics, economics, business, psychology, education, and many other natural, biological, and social sciences. The JSS Series of Statistics aims to publish recent results of current research activities in the areas of statistics and statistical sciences in Japan that otherwise would not be available in English; they are complementary to the two JSS academic journals, both English and Japanese. Because the scope of a research paper in academic journals inevitably has become narrowly focused and condensed in recent years, this series is intended to fill the gap between academic research activities and the form of a single academic paper. The series will be of great interest to a wide audience of researchers, teachers, professional statisticians, and graduate students in many countries who are interested in statistics and statistical sciences, in statistical theory, and in various areas of statistical applications.

More information about this subseries at https://link.springer.com/bookseries/13497

Taka-aki Shiraishi

Multiple Comparisons
for Bernoulli Data

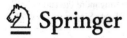 Springer

Taka-aki Shiraishi
Faculty of Science and Technology
Nanzan University
Nagoya, Aichi, Japan

ISSN 2191-544X   ISSN 2191-5458 (electronic)
SpringerBriefs in Statistics
ISSN 2364-0057   ISSN 2364-0065 (electronic)
JSS Research Series in Statistics
ISBN 978-981-19-2707-2   ISBN 978-981-19-2708-9 (eBook)
https://doi.org/10.1007/978-981-19-2708-9

This Springer imprint is published by the registered company Springer Nature Singapore Pte Ltd.
The registered company address is: 152 Beach Road, #21-01/04 Gateway East, Singapore 189721,
Singapore

Preface

Multiple tests and simultaneous confidence intervals specify differences in means. Tukey (1953), Miller (1981), Hochberg and Tamhane (1987), Hsu (1996), and Shiraishi et al. (2018), (2019) are some technical books on multiple comparisons for continuous random variables. Multiple comparisons for discrete random variables have been discussed a little. The present book focuses on progressive multiple comparisons of proportions in multi-sample models with Bernoulli responses.

In Chap. 1, we give theoretical basics in one-sample and two-sample models. We state regurarity conditions of exact confidence limit using F-distribution. We introduce asymptotic theory based on variance-stabilizing transformation. In Chap. 2, we give simultaneous inference for all proportions in multi-sample models by using the exact confidence limit and the asymptotic theory. In Chap. 3, we discuss all-pairwise multiple comparison tests of proportions. Closed testing procedures based on maximum absolute values of some two-sample test statistics and based on χ^2-test statistics are introduced in multi-sample models. The results suggest that the multi-step procedures are more effective than single-step procedures and the Ryan–Einot–Gabriel–Welsch (REGW) type tests. In Chap. 4, we give multiple comparison test procedures with a control. In Chap. 5, we propose simultaneous confidence intervals for difference of proportions, odds ratio, and ratio of proportions. By the theory of this intervals, we are able to obtain all-pairwise multiple comparison tests of odds ratio. In Chaps. 6 and 7, under simple ordered restrictions of proportions, we also discuss closed testing procedures based on maximum values of two-sample one-sided test statistics and based on Bartholomew's $\bar{\chi}^2$-statistics. Although single-step multiple comparison procedures are utilized in general, the closed testing procedures stated in the present book are fairly more powerful than the single-step procedures. Bretz et al. (2011) discuss serial gatekeeping methods based on Bonferroni inequality.

In Chaps. 8 and 9, we propose serial gatekeeping methods based on the closed testing procedures stated in Chaps. 3, 4, 6 and 7. It is shown that the proposed serial gatekeeping methods are much superior to the serial gatekeeping methods based on Bonferroni tests.

Nagoya, Japan   Taka-aki Shiraishi
March 2022

References

Bretz F, Hothorn T, Westfall P (2010) Multiple comparisons using R. Chapman & Hall

Hochberg Y, Tamhane AC (1987) Multiple comparison procedures. Wiley

Hsu JC (1996) Multiple comparisons-theory and methods. Chapman & Hall

Miller RG (1981) Simultaneous statistical inference, 2rd edn. Springer

Shiraishi T, Sugiura H (2018) Theory of multiple comparison procedures and its computation. Kyoritsu-Shuppan Co., Ltd. (in Japanese)

Shiraishi T, Sugiura H, Matsuda S (2019) Pairwise multiple comparisons-theory and computation. SpringerBriefs. Springer International Publishing

Tukey JW (1953). The problem of multiple comparisons. The Collected Works of John W. Tukey (1994), Volume VIII: Multiple Comparisons. Chapman & Hall

Acknowledgements

The authors are grateful to two referees for valuable comments. This research was supported in part by a Grant-in-Aid for Co-operative Research (C) 18K11204 from the Japanese Ministry of Education. This research was also supported in part by Nanzan University Pache Research Subsidy I-A-2 for 2021 academic year.

Contents

Chapter 1
Theoretical Basics in One-Sample and Two-Sample Models

Abstract Before discussing multiple comparisons of the multi-sample Bernoulli models, we state the basics of statistics in the one-sample and two-sample models. As for the method related to the Bernoulli model, a method called exact confidence limit using the F distribution is introduced in the statistics. The regularity conditions that have been overlooked so far are added. Furthermore, for large sample theory, the method based on the variance-stabilizing transformation is described.

1.1 Exact Theory in One-Sample Model

We suppose specifically that $(X_1, \ldots, X_n)$ is a random sample of size n from the Bernoulli population with success probability p. It is convenient to assign the number 1 to a success and the number 0 to a failure.

$$P(X_i = 1) = p \text{ and } P(X_i = 0) = 1 - p$$

hold. X_i's are assumed to be independent. The number of successes is given by

$$X := X_1 + \ldots + X_n. \tag{1.1}$$

For $x = 0, 1, \ldots, n$, the frequency function of X is given by

$$f(x|n, p) := P(X = x) = \binom{n}{x} p^x (1 - p)^{n-x}. \tag{1.2}$$

The random variable X has a binomial distribution $B(n, p)$. The mean and variance of X are given by

$$E(X) = np \text{ and } V(X) = np(1 - p),$$

© The Author(s), under exclusive license to Springer Nature Singapore Pte Ltd. 2022 1
T. Shiraishi, *Multiple Comparisons for Bernoulli Data*,
JSS Research Series in Statistics,
https://doi.org/10.1007/978-981-19-2708-9_1

respectively. If the parameter p is 0 or 1, the statistical inference is trivial. Henceforth we assume

$$0 < p < 1. \tag{1.3}$$

We get Lemma 1.1.

Lemma 1.1 *Suppose that X has a binomial distribution $B(n, p)$. For positive integers m_1 and m_2, let $\mathscr{F}_{m_2}^{m_1}$ be a random variable having F-distribution with m_1 and m_2 degrees of freedom. Then we get, for $x = 0, 1, \ldots, n$,*

$$P(X \geq x) = P\left(\mathscr{F}_{2x}^{2(n-x+1)} \geq \frac{x(1-p)}{(n-x+1)p}\right), \tag{1.4}$$

and

$$P(X \leq x) = P\left(\mathscr{F}_{2(n-x)}^{2(x+1)} \geq \frac{(n-x)p}{(x+1)(1-p)}\right) \tag{1.5}$$

where $\mathscr{F}_0^m = 1$ for positive integer m. Furthermore the upper probability $P(X \geq x)$ is a increasing function in p and the lower probability $P(X \leq x)$ is a decreasing function in p.

Proof Refer to Lemma 7.5 of Shiraishi (2012). □

For $f(x|n, p)$ of (1.2) and α satisfying $0 < \alpha < 1$, we add the condition (c.1).

$$p^n \leq \alpha \quad (\Longleftrightarrow \ p \leq \alpha^{1/n}). \tag{c.1}$$

We define $u(p, n; \alpha)$ by a minimal positive integer that satisfies

$$P(X \geq u(p, n; \alpha)) = \sum_{j=u(p,n;\alpha)}^{n} f(j|n, p) \leq \alpha. \tag{1.6}$$

From (1.4), we can give the value of $u(p, n; \alpha)$. From Lemma 1.1, we find that $F(x|n, p)$ is continuous and decreasing in p. We add the condition (c.2).

$$(1-p)^n \leq \alpha \quad (\Longleftrightarrow \ p \geq 1 - \alpha^{1/n}). \tag{c.2}$$

We define $\ell(p, n; \alpha)$ by a maximal integer that satisfies

$$P(X \leq \ell(p, n; \alpha)) = \sum_{j=0}^{\ell(p,n;\alpha)} f(j|n, p) \leq \alpha.$$

From (1.5), we can give the value of $\ell(p, n; \alpha)$. From the second half assertion of Lemma 1.1, $u(p, n; \alpha)$ and $\ell(p, n; \alpha)$ are increasing in p. We get Theorem 1.1.

Theorem 1.1 *For positive integers m_1 and m_2, let $F_{m_2}^{m_1}(\alpha)$ be an upper $100\alpha\%$ point of F-distribution with m_1 and m_2 degrees of freedom. Then, under the condition (c.1), for X of (1.1),*

$$\{X \geq u(p, n; \alpha)\} = \left\{ p \leq \frac{L}{K \cdot F_L^K(\alpha) + L} \right\} \tag{1.7}$$

holds, where $F_0^m(\alpha) = 1$, and random variables K and L are defined by

$$K := 2(n - X + 1) \ and \ L := 2X. \tag{1.8}$$

Furthermore, under the condition (c.2),

$$\{X \leq \ell(p, n; \alpha)\} = \left\{ p \geq \frac{K^* \cdot F_{L^*}^{K^*}(\alpha)}{K^* \cdot F_{L^*}^{K^*}(\alpha) + L^*} \right\} \tag{1.9}$$

holds, where random variables K^* and L^* are defined by

$$K^* := 2(X + 1) \ and \ L^* := 2(n - X). \tag{1.10}$$

Proof If (c.1) does not hold, there does not exist $u(p, n; \alpha)$ satisfying the inequality of the right-hand side of (1.6). Let x be a nonnegative integer such that

$$x < u(p, n; \alpha). \tag{1.11}$$

Then from (1.4) of Lemma 1.1, (1.11) is equivalent to

$$P\left(F_{2x}^{2(n-x+1)} \geq \frac{x(1-p)}{(n-x+1)p} \right) = \sum_{j=x}^{n} f(j|n, p) > \alpha. \tag{1.12}$$

Furthermore (1.12) is equivalent to

$$F_{2x}^{2(n-x+1)}(\alpha) > \frac{x(1-p)}{(n-x+1)p} \iff p > \frac{2x}{2(n-x+1)F_{2x}^{2(n-x+1)}(\alpha) + 2x}.$$

Hence we have

$$\left\{ \omega \middle| X(\omega) < u(p, n; \alpha) \right\} = \left\{ \omega \middle| p > \frac{L(\omega)}{K(\omega) \cdot F_{L(\omega)}^{K(\omega)}(\alpha) + L(\omega)} \right\}.$$

By taking the complementary events on both sides of the above equation, we get

$$\{\omega \mid X(\omega) \geq u(p, n; \alpha)\} = \left\{\omega \;\middle|\; p \leq \frac{L(\omega)}{K(\omega) \cdot F_{L(\omega)}^{K(\omega)}(\alpha) + L(\omega)}\right\}. \tag{1.13}$$

This fact implies (1.7). Similarly, we get (1.9). □

From Theorem 1.1, we get Corollary 1.1.

Corollary 1.1 *Under (c.1),*

$$P\left(\frac{L}{K \cdot F_L^K(\alpha) + L} \geq p\right) = P(X \geq u(p, n; \alpha)) \leq \alpha \tag{1.14}$$

holds and, under (c.2),

$$P\left(\frac{K^* \cdot F_{L^*}^{K^*}(\alpha)}{K^* \cdot F_{L^*}^{K^*}(\alpha) + L^*} \leq p\right) = P(X \leq \ell(p, n; \alpha)) \leq \alpha \tag{1.15}$$

holds. □

Let us put

$$A := \left\{\frac{L}{K \cdot F_L^K(\frac{\alpha}{2}) + L} \geq p\right\}, \quad B := \left\{\frac{K^* \cdot F_{L^*}^{K^*}(\frac{\alpha}{2})}{K^* \cdot F_{L^*}^{K^*}(\frac{\alpha}{2}) + L^*} \leq p\right\}.$$

Then since $\alpha/2 < 0.5$, from Corollary 1.1, we get $A \cap B = \emptyset$. Hence

$$P(A \cup B) = P(A) + P(B) \leq \alpha \tag{1.16}$$

holds.

We give a constant p_0 such that $0 < p_0 < 1$. We consider three sorts of the following hypotheses.

① the null hypothesis $H_1 : p = p_0$ versus the alternative $H_1^A : p \neq p_0$
② the null hypothesis $H_2 : p \leq p_0$ versus the alternative $H_2^A : p > p_0$
③ the null hypothesis $H_3 : p \geq p_0$ versus the alternative $H_3^A : p < p_0$.

From (1.7), (1.9) and (1.16) of Theorem 1.1, we have the test procedures of [1.1].

[1.1] Exact Conservative Tests
The test procedures are given by (1)–(3) for ① – ③.

(1) The two conditions of $p_0^n \leq \alpha/2$ and $(1 - p_0)^n \leq \alpha/2$ are added. Whenever

$$\frac{L}{K F_L^K\left(\frac{\alpha}{2}\right) + L} \geq p_0 \quad \text{or} \quad \frac{K^* F_{L^*}^{K^*}\left(\frac{\alpha}{2}\right)}{K^* F_{L^*}^{K^*}\left(\frac{\alpha}{2}\right) + L^*} \leq p_0$$

holds, we reject the null hypothesis H_1 as a test of level α for the null hypothesis H_1 versus the alternative H_1^A.

(2) The condition of $p_0^n \leq \alpha$ is added. Whenever

$$\frac{L}{K F_L^K (\alpha) + L} \geq p_0$$

holds, we reject the null hypothesis H_2 as a test of level α for the null hypothesis H_2 versus the alternative H_2^A.

(3) The condition of $(1 - p_0)^n \leq \alpha$ is added. Whenever

$$\frac{K^* F_{L^*}^{K^*} (\alpha)}{K^* F_{L^*}^{K^*} (\alpha) + L^*} \leq p_0$$

holds, we reject the null hypothesis H_3 as a test of level α for the null hypothesis H_3 versus the alternative H_3^A.

Since, for $p \leq p_0$,

$$P \left(\frac{L}{K \cdot F_L^K (\alpha) + L} \geq p_0 \right) \leq P \left(\frac{L}{K \cdot F_L^K (\alpha) + L} \geq p \right) \leq \alpha$$

holds, we find that the size of the above test (2) is α. The size of the above test (3) is also α.

The test procedure of (1) is given by the test function

$$\phi(X) = \begin{cases} 1 \left(\frac{L}{K F_L^K (\frac{\alpha}{2})+L} \geq p_0 \text{ or } \frac{K^* F_{L^*}^{K^*} (\frac{\alpha}{2})}{K^* F_{L^*}^{K^*} (\frac{\alpha}{2})+L^*} \leq p_0 \right) \\ 0 \left(\frac{L}{K F_L^K (\frac{\alpha}{2})+L} < p_0 < \frac{K^* F_{L^*}^{K^*} (\frac{\alpha}{2})}{K^* F_{L^*}^{K^*} (\frac{\alpha}{2})+L^*} \right). \end{cases} \tag{1.17}$$

From (1.7) and (1.9) of Theorem 1.1, we find that (1.17) is equivalent to

$$\phi(X) = \begin{cases} 1 \ (X \leq \ell(p_0, n; \alpha/2) \text{ or } X \geq u(p_0, n; \alpha/2)) \\ 0 \ (\ell(p_0, n; \alpha/2) + 1 \leq X \leq u(p_0, n; \alpha/2) - 1). \end{cases} \tag{1.18}$$

[1.2] Exact Tests
We propose the test of

$$\phi(X) = \begin{cases} 1 \ (X \geq u(p_0, n; \alpha/2) \text{ or } X \leq \ell(p_0, n; \alpha/2)) \\ \gamma_1 \ (X = u(p_0, n; \alpha/2) - 1) \\ \gamma_2 \ (X = \ell(p_0, n; \alpha/2) + 1) \\ 0 \ (\ell(p_0, n; \alpha/2) + 1 < X < u(p_0, n; \alpha/2) - 1), \end{cases} \tag{1.19}$$

where

$$\gamma_1 := \frac{\alpha/2 - P_0 \left(X \geq u(p_0, n; \alpha/2) \right)}{P_0 \left(X = u(p_0, n; \alpha/2) - 1 \right)} \text{ and } \gamma_2 := \frac{\alpha/2 - P_0 \left(X \leq \ell(p_0, n; \alpha/2) \right)}{P_0 \left(X = \ell(p_0, n; \alpha/2) + 1 \right)}$$

and $P_0(\cdot)$ stands for probability measure under H_1. Since, under the null hypothesis H_1, $E\{\phi(X)\} = \alpha$ holds, (1.19) is a test of level α. The values of γ_1 and γ_2 are given by using (1.4) and (1.5).

The power of the test (1.19) is higher than the test (1.18).

Under the condition of $p_0^n \leq \alpha$, for the null hypothesis H_2 versus the alternative H_2^A, we propose the test procedure given by the test function

$$\phi(X) = \begin{cases} 1 & (X \geq u(p_0, n; \alpha)) \\ \gamma & (X = u(p_0, n; \alpha) - 1) \\ 0 & (X < u(p_0, n; \alpha) - 1), \end{cases} \tag{1.20}$$

where

$$\gamma := \frac{\alpha - P_0\left(X \geq u(p_0, n; \alpha)\right)}{P_0\left(X = u(p_0, n; \alpha) - 1\right)}.$$

We get Proposition 1.1.

Proposition 1.1 *The procedure of (1.20) is a test of level α.*

Proof We suppose $p \leq p_0$. We have

$$E\{\phi(X)\} = P(X \geq u(p_0, n; \alpha)) + \gamma P(X = u(p_0, n; \alpha) - 1)$$
$$= \gamma P(X \geq u(p_0, n; \alpha) - 1) + (1 - \gamma)P(X \geq u(p_0, n; \alpha)).$$

From this fact and the second half assertion of Lemma 1.1, we get

$$E\{\phi(X)\} \leq E_0\{\phi(X)\} = \alpha,$$

where $E_0(\cdot)$ denote the expectation under $p = p_0$. Hence we get the assertion. □

Under the condition of $(1 - p_0)^n \leq \alpha$, for the null hypothesis H_3 versus the alternative H_3^A, we propose the test procedure given by the test function

$$\phi(X) = \begin{cases} 1 & (X \leq \ell(p_0, n; \alpha)) \\ \frac{\alpha - P_0(X \leq \ell(p_0, n; \alpha))}{P_0(X = \ell(p_0, n; \alpha) + 1)} & (X = \ell(p_0, n; \alpha) + 1) \\ 0 & (X > \ell(p_0, n; \alpha) + 1). \end{cases}$$

From Corollary 1.1, we get Theorem 1.2.

Theorem 1.2 *Suppose that $p^n \leq \alpha/2$ and $(1 - p)^n \leq \alpha/2$ are satisfied. Then*

$$P\left(\frac{L}{K F_L^K\left(\frac{\alpha}{2}\right) + L} < p < \frac{K^* F_{L^*}^{K^*}\left(\frac{\alpha}{2}\right)}{K^* F_{L^*}^{K^*}\left(\frac{\alpha}{2}\right) + L^*}\right) \geq 1 - \alpha$$

holds.   □

From Corollary 1.1 and Theorem 1.2, we have confidence intervals and bounds of [1.3].

[1.3] Exact Conservative Confidence Interval and Bounds for Proportion
The confidence interval and bounds for p are expressed by (1)–(3).

(1) Under the conditions of $p^n \leq \alpha/2$ and $(1-p)^n \leq \alpha/2$, the $100(1-\alpha)\%$ confidence interval for p is given by

$$\frac{L}{KF_L^K\left(\frac{\alpha}{2}\right)+L} < p < \frac{K^*F_{L^*}^{K^*}\left(\frac{\alpha}{2}\right)}{K^*F_{L^*}^{K^*}\left(\frac{\alpha}{2}\right)+L^*}.$$

(2) Under the condition (c.1), the $100(1-\alpha)\%$ lower confidence bound for p is given by

$$\frac{L}{KF_L^K(\alpha)+L} < p < 1.$$

(3) Under the condition (c.2), the $100(1-\alpha)\%$ upper confidence bound for p is given by

$$0 < p < \frac{K^*F_{L^*}^{K^*}(\alpha)}{K^*F_{L^*}^{K^*}(\alpha)+L^*}.$$

(1) of [1.3] is given by Clopper and Pearson (1934).

The odds ratio $g(p) := p/(1-p)$ is strictly increasing in p. From [1.3], we have confidence interval and bounds of [1.4] for odds ratio.

[1.4] Exact Conservative Confidence Interval and Bounds for Odds Ratio
The confidence interval and bounds for $p/(1-p)$ are expressed by (1)–(3).

(1) Under the conditions of $p^n \leq \alpha/2$ and $(1-p)^n \leq \alpha/2$, the $100(1-\alpha)\%$ confidence interval for $p/(1-p)$ is given by

$$\frac{L}{KF_L^K\left(\frac{\alpha}{2}\right)} < \frac{p}{1-p} < \frac{K^*F_{L^*}^{K^*}\left(\frac{\alpha}{2}\right)}{L^*}.$$

(2) Under the condition (c.1), the $100(1-\alpha)\%$ lower confidence bound for $p/(1-p)$ is given by

$$\frac{L}{KF_L^K(\alpha)} < \frac{p}{1-p} < \infty.$$

(3) Under the condition (c.2), the $100(1-\alpha)\%$ upper confidence bound for $p/(1-p)$ is given by

$$0 < \frac{p}{1-p} < \frac{K^*F_{L^*}^{K^*}(\alpha)}{L^*}.$$

1.2   Asymptotic Theory in One-Sample Model

We discuss asymptotic procedures. For X of (1.1), the estimator of p is given by

$$\hat{p} := \frac{X}{n} \quad \text{or} \quad \frac{X + 0.5}{n + 1}. \tag{1.21}$$

We have $E(X_i) = p$ and $V(X_i) = p(1 - p)$. It follows that, from a central limit theorem, as $n \to \infty$,

$$\frac{\sqrt{n}(\hat{p} - p)}{\sqrt{p(1 - p)}} \xrightarrow{\mathscr{L}} Z \sim N(0, 1) \tag{1.22}$$

holds, where $\xrightarrow{\mathscr{L}}$ denotes convergence in law. Furthermore, we have

$$\frac{d}{dx} \arcsin\left(\sqrt{x}\right) = \frac{1}{2\sqrt{x(1 - x)}}. \tag{1.23}$$

Hence from (1.22) and (1.23), by using Slutsky's theorem and delta method, we get

$$\sqrt{n}\left\{\arcsin\left(\sqrt{\hat{p}}\right) - \arcsin\left(\sqrt{p}\right)\right\} \xrightarrow{\mathscr{L}} N\left(0, \frac{1}{4}\right). \tag{1.24}$$

Let us put

$$T_1 := 2\sqrt{n}\left\{\arcsin\left(\sqrt{\hat{p}}\right) - \arcsin\left(\sqrt{p_0}\right)\right\} \quad \text{or} \quad \frac{\sqrt{n}(\hat{p} - p_0)}{\sqrt{\hat{p}(1 - \hat{p})}}.$$

Then, from (1.22) and (1.24), we find

$$\lim_{n \to \infty} P_0(|T_1| > z(\alpha/2)) = P(|Z| > z(\alpha/2)) = \alpha, \tag{1.25}$$

where $z(\alpha)$ stands for the upper $100\alpha\%$ point of the standard normal distribution.
From (1.25), we have the test procedure of [1.5].

[1.5] Two-Sided Test
By using test function $\phi(\cdot)$, an asymptotic test of level α for the null hypothesis H_1 versus the alternative H_1^A is given by

$$\phi(X) = \begin{cases} 1 & (|T_1| > z(\alpha/2)) \\ 0 & (|T_1| < z(\alpha/2)). \end{cases}$$

Similarly, we are able to give asymptotic one-sided tests of level α.
From (1.22), we have

$$\lim_{n \to \infty} P\left(\left| \frac{\sqrt{n}(\hat{p} - p)}{\sqrt{p(1 - p)}} \right| < z(\alpha/2) \right) = 1 - \alpha.$$

We find that

$$\left| \frac{\sqrt{n}(\hat{p} - p)}{\sqrt{p(1 - p)}} \right|^2 < z^2(\alpha/2)$$

is equivalent to

$$\frac{2n\hat{p} + z^2(\alpha/2) - \sqrt{4nz^2(\alpha/2)\hat{p}(1 - \hat{p}) + z^4(\alpha/2)}}{2(n + z^2(\alpha/2))}$$
$$< p < \frac{2n\hat{p} + z^2(\alpha/2) + \sqrt{4nz^2(\alpha/2)\hat{p}(1 - \hat{p}) + z^4(\alpha/2)}}{2(n + z^2(\alpha/2))}. \tag{1.26}$$

Hence (1.26) is a $100(1 - \alpha)\%$ asymptotic confidence interval for p.

Since, from (1.22) and (1.24), we get

$$\lim_{n \to \infty} P\left(\left| \frac{\sqrt{n}(\hat{p} - p)}{\sqrt{\hat{p}(1 - \hat{p})}} \right| < z(\alpha/2) \right) = 1 - \alpha$$

and

$$\lim_{n \to \infty} P\left(\left| 2\sqrt{n} \left\{ \arcsin\left(\sqrt{\hat{p}} \right) - \arcsin\left(\sqrt{p} \right) \right\} \right| < z(\alpha/2) \right) = 1 - \alpha,$$

we find that

$$\hat{p} - z(\alpha/2) \cdot \sqrt{\frac{\hat{p}(1 - \hat{p})}{n}} < p < \hat{p} + z(\alpha/2) \cdot \sqrt{\frac{\hat{p}(1 - \hat{p})}{n}} \tag{1.27}$$

and

$$\sin^2\left[\max\left\{ \arcsin\left(\sqrt{\hat{p}} \right) - \frac{z(\alpha/2)}{2\sqrt{n}}, 0 \right\} \right]$$
$$< p < \sin^2\left[\min\left\{ \arcsin\left(\sqrt{\hat{p}} \right) + \frac{z(\alpha/2)}{2\sqrt{n}}, \frac{\pi}{2} \right\} \right] \tag{1.28}$$

are also a $100(1 - \alpha)\%$ asymptotic confidence interval for p.

The confidence intervals of (1.27) and (1.26) may contain 0 or 1. Hence we consider logit transformations

$$\theta := \log\left(\frac{p}{1 - p} \right) \iff p = \frac{e^\theta}{e^\theta + 1} \tag{1.29}$$

and

$$\hat{\theta} := \log\left(\frac{\hat{p}}{1-\hat{p}}\right).$$

We put

$$c := \frac{d\theta}{dp} = \frac{1}{p} + \frac{1}{1-p} = \frac{1}{p(1-p)}. \tag{1.30}$$

From the delta method, (1.22) and (1.30), we have

$$\sqrt{n}(\hat{\theta} - \theta) \overset{\mathcal{L}}{\to} c\sqrt{p(1-p)}Z \sim N\left(0, \frac{1}{p(1-p)}\right), \tag{1.31}$$

which implies

$$\lim_{n\to\infty} P\left(\sqrt{n\hat{p}(1-\hat{p})} \cdot |\hat{\theta} - \theta| < z(\alpha/2)\right) = 1 - \alpha.$$

Hence a $100(1-\alpha)\%$ asymptotic confidence intervals for θ is given by

$$\hat{\theta} - z(\alpha/2)/\sqrt{n\hat{p}(1-\hat{p})} < \theta < \hat{\theta} + z(\alpha/2)/\sqrt{n\hat{p}(1-\hat{p})}.$$

From (1.29), we get Theorem 1.3.

Theorem 1.3

$$\lim_{n\to\infty} P\left(\frac{\exp\left(\hat{\theta} - z(\alpha/2) \cdot SD_n\right)}{\exp\left(\hat{\theta} - z(\alpha/2) \cdot SD_n\right) + 1} < p < \frac{\exp\left(\hat{\theta} + z(\alpha/2) \cdot SD_n\right)}{\exp\left(\hat{\theta} + z(\alpha/2) \cdot SD_n\right) + 1}\right)$$

$$= 1 - \alpha$$

holds, where

$$SD_n := \frac{1}{\sqrt{n\hat{p}(1-\hat{p})}}. \tag{1.32}$$

$\square$

From Theorem 1.3 and similar discussion, we derive asymptotic confidence interval and bounds of [1.6].

[1.6] Asymptotic Confidence Interval and Bounds
The asymptotic confidence interval and bounds for p are expressed by (1)–(3).

(1) The $100(1-\alpha)\%$ asymptotic confidence interval for p is given by

$$\frac{\exp\left(\hat{\theta} - z(\alpha/2) \cdot SD_n\right)}{\exp\left(\hat{\theta} - z(\alpha/2) \cdot SD_n\right) + 1} < p < \frac{\exp\left(\hat{\theta} + z(\alpha/2) \cdot SD_n\right)}{\exp\left(\hat{\theta} + z(\alpha/2) \cdot SD_n\right) + 1},$$

where SD_n is defined by (1.32).

(2) The $100(1 - \alpha)\%$ asymptotic lower confidence bound for p is given by

$$\frac{\exp\left(\hat{\theta} - z(\alpha) \cdot SD_n\right)}{\exp\left(\hat{\theta} - z(\alpha) \cdot SD_n\right) + 1} < p < 1.$$

(3) The $100(1 - \alpha)\%$ asymptotic upper confidence bound for p is given by

$$0 < p < \frac{\exp\left(\hat{\theta} + z(\alpha) \cdot SD_n\right)}{\exp\left(\hat{\theta} + z(\alpha) \cdot SD_n\right) + 1}.$$

These confidence intervals do not contain 0 and 1.

1.3   Asymptotic Theory in Two-Sample Model

We suppose that $(X_1, \ldots, X_{n_1})$ is a random sample of size n_1 from the Bernoulli population with success probability p_1 and $(Y_1, \ldots, Y_{n_2})$ is a random sample of size n_2 from the Bernoulli population with success probability p_2. Furthermore we suppose that $(X_1, \ldots, X_{n_1})$ and $(Y_1, \ldots, Y_{n_2})$ are independent. Thereafter we assume $0 < p_i < 1$ $(i = 1, 2)$. We put

$$X := X_1 + \ldots + X_{n_1}, \quad Y := Y_1 + \ldots + Y_{n_2},$$

$$\hat{p}_1 := \frac{X}{n_1} \text{ or } \frac{X + 0.5}{n_1 + 1}, \quad \hat{p}_2 := \frac{Y}{n_2} \text{ or } \frac{Y + 0.5}{n_2 + 1} \text{ and } n := n_1 + n_2.$$

We add the condition (c.3)

$$0 < \lim_{n \to \infty} \frac{n_1}{n} = \lambda < 1. \tag{c.3}$$

By the way similar to (1.22), we get

$$\sqrt{n}(\hat{p}_1 - p_1) \overset{\mathscr{L}}{\to} \sqrt{\frac{p_1(1 - p_1)}{\lambda}} \cdot Z_1 \tag{1.33}$$

and

$$\sqrt{n}(\hat{p}_2 - p_2) \overset{\mathscr{L}}{\to} \sqrt{\frac{p_2(1 - p_2)}{1 - \lambda}} \cdot Z_2, \tag{1.34}$$

where Z_1 and Z_2 stand for independent standard normal random variables.

From (1.23), (1.33), and (1.34), by using Slutsky's theorem and delta method, we get

$$\sqrt{n} \left\{ \arcsin \left(\sqrt{\hat{p}_1} \right) - \arcsin \left(\sqrt{p_1} \right) \right\} \overset{\mathscr{L}}{\to} \tilde{Z}_1 \sim N \left(0, \frac{1}{4\lambda} \right) \tag{1.35}$$

and

$$\sqrt{n} \left\{ \arcsin \left(\sqrt{\hat{p}_2} \right) - \arcsin \left(\sqrt{p_2} \right) \right\} \overset{\mathscr{L}}{\to} \tilde{Z}_2 \sim N \left(0, \frac{1}{4(1-\lambda)} \right). \tag{1.36}$$

For the null hypothesis $H_0 : p_1 = p_2$, we consider three sorts of the following alternative hypotheses (i)–(iii).

$$\text{(i) } H_1^A : p_1 \neq p_2 \quad \text{(ii) } H_2^A : p_1 > p_2 \quad \text{(iii) } H_3^A : p_1 < p_2.$$

Let us put

$$T_2 := \frac{2 \left\{ \arcsin \left(\sqrt{\hat{p}_1} \right) - \arcsin \left(\sqrt{\hat{p}_2} \right) \right\}}{\sqrt{\frac{1}{n_1} + \frac{1}{n_2}}} \quad \text{or} \quad \frac{\hat{p}_1 - \hat{p}_2}{\tilde{\sigma}_n},$$

where

$$\tilde{\sigma}_n := \sqrt{\frac{1}{n_1} \hat{p}_1 (1 - \hat{p}_1) + \frac{1}{n_2} \hat{p}_2 (1 - \hat{p}_2)}.$$

Then from (1.33)–(1.36), under H_0, we find

$$T_2 \overset{\mathscr{L}}{\to} N(0, 1).$$

Hence we have the test procedures of [1.7].

[1.7] Asymptotic Tests

The test procedures are given by (1)–(3) for the alternative hypotheses of (i)-(iii).

(1) Whenever $|T_2| > z(\alpha/2)$ holds, we reject the null hypothesis H_0 as a test of level α for the null hypothesis H_0 versus the alternative H_1^A.

(2) Whenever $T_2 > z(\alpha)$ holds, we reject the null hypothesis H_0 as a test of level α for the null hypothesis H_0 versus the alternative H_2^A.

(3) Whenever $-T_2 > z(\alpha)$ holds, we reject the null hypothesis H_0 as a test of level α for the null hypothesis H_0 versus the alternative H_3^A.

From (1.33) and (1.34), we have

$$\frac{\hat{p}_1 - \hat{p}_2 - p_1 + p_2}{\tilde{\sigma}_n} \overset{\mathscr{L}}{\to} N(0, 1).$$

Hence the $100(1 - \alpha)\%$ asymptotic confidence interval for $p_1 - p_2$ is given by

$$p_1 - p_2 \in \hat{p}_1 - \hat{p}_2 \pm z(\alpha/2) \cdot \tilde{\sigma}_n. \tag{1.37}$$

If we put

$$\hat{p}_1 = \frac{X}{n_1} \text{ and } \hat{p}_2 = \frac{Y}{n_2}, \tag{1.38}$$

Interval (1.37) is equivalent to

$$p_1 - p_2 \in \frac{X}{n_1} - \frac{Y}{n_2} \pm z(\alpha/2) \cdot \sqrt{\frac{X(n_1 - X)}{n_1^3} + \frac{Y(n_2 - Y)}{n_2^3}}. \tag{1.39}$$

Interval (1.39) is appeared in Daniel (1987). The relation of $-1 < p_1 - p_2 < 1$ is satisfied. However the confidence interval of (1.39) may contain 1 or -1. Thus we consider logit transformation

$$\theta := \log\left(\frac{\frac{p_1 - p_2 + 1}{2}}{1 - \frac{p_1 - p_2 + 1}{2}}\right) = \log\left\{\frac{p_1 - p_2 + 1}{1 - (p_1 - p_2)}\right\},$$

which implies

$$p_1 - p_2 = \frac{e^\theta - 1}{e^\theta + 1}. \tag{1.40}$$

We put

$$c := \frac{d\theta}{d(p_1 - p_2)} = \frac{1}{1 + p_1 - p_2} + \frac{1}{1 - (p_1 - p_2)} = \frac{2}{1 - (p_1 - p_2)^2}. \tag{1.41}$$

Furthermore let us put

$$\hat{\theta} := \log\left\{\frac{\hat{p}_1 - \hat{p}_2 + 1}{1 - (\hat{p}_1 - \hat{p}_2)}\right\}.$$

Then, from (1.33) and (1.34), we get

$$\sqrt{n}(\hat{p}_1 - \hat{p}_2 - p_1 + p_2) \xrightarrow{\mathscr{L}} \sqrt{\frac{p_1(1 - p_1)}{\lambda}} \cdot Z_1 - \sqrt{\frac{p_2(1 - p_2)}{1 - \lambda}} \cdot Z_2. \tag{1.42}$$

By applying $h(x) := \log\{(x + 1)/(1 - x)\}$ in Theorem 5.3.3 (delta method) of Bickel and Doksum (2001), (1.41) and (1.42) give

$$\sqrt{n}(\hat{\theta} - \theta) \xrightarrow{\mathcal{L}} c \left(\sqrt{\frac{p_1(1 - p_1)}{\lambda}} \cdot Z_1 - \sqrt{\frac{p_2(1 - p_2)}{1 - \lambda}} \cdot Z_2 \right)$$

$$\sim N\left(0, \frac{c^2 p_1(1 - p_1)}{\lambda} + \frac{c^2 p_2(1 - p_2)}{1 - \lambda} \right). \tag{1.43}$$

Let us put

$$SD_n := \frac{2}{1 - (\hat{p}_1 - \hat{p}_2)^2} \cdot \sqrt{\frac{1}{n_1} \hat{p}_1(1 - \hat{p}_1) + \frac{1}{n_2} \hat{p}_2(1 - \hat{p}_2)}. \tag{1.44}$$

Then (1.43) gives

$$\frac{\hat{\theta} - \theta}{SD_n} \xrightarrow{\mathcal{L}} N(0, 1).$$

Hence the $100(1 - \alpha)\%$ asymptotic confidence interval for θ is given by

$$\hat{\theta} - z(\alpha/2) \cdot SD_n < \theta < \hat{\theta} + z(\alpha/2) \cdot SD_n.$$

From (1.40), we derive asymptotic confidence interval and bounds of [1.8] for $p_1 - p_2$.

[1.8] Asymptotic Confidence Interval and Bounds

The asymptotic confidence interval and bounds for $p_1 - p_2$ are expressed by (1)–(3).

(1) The $100(1 - \alpha)\%$ asymptotic confidence interval for $p_1 - p_2$ is given by

$$\frac{\exp(\hat{\theta} - z(\alpha/2) \cdot SD_n) - 1}{\exp(\hat{\theta} - z(\alpha/2) \cdot SD_n) + 1} < p_1 - p_2 < \frac{\exp(\hat{\theta} + z(\alpha/2) \cdot SD_n) - 1}{\exp(\hat{\theta} + z(\alpha/2) \cdot SD_n) + 1},$$

where SD_n is defined by (1.44).

(2) The $100(1 - \alpha)\%$ asymptotic lower confidence bound for $p_1 - p_2$ is given by

$$\frac{\exp(\hat{\theta} - z(\alpha) \cdot SD_n) - 1}{\exp(\hat{\theta} - z(\alpha) \cdot SD_n) + 1} < p_1 - p_2 < 1.$$

(3) The $100(1 - \alpha)\%$ asymptotic upper confidence bound for $p_1 - p_2$ is given by

$$-1 < p_1 - p_2 < \frac{\exp(\hat{\theta} + z(\alpha) \cdot SD_n) - 1}{\exp(\hat{\theta} + z(\alpha) \cdot SD_n) + 1}.$$

Equations (1.35) and (1.36) imply

$$\frac{2\left\{\arcsin\left(\sqrt{\hat{p}_1}\right) - \arcsin\left(\sqrt{\hat{p}_2}\right) - \arcsin\left(\sqrt{p_1}\right) + \arcsin\left(\sqrt{p_2}\right)\right\}}{\sqrt{\frac{1}{n_1} + \frac{1}{n_2}}} \xrightarrow{\mathscr{L}} N(0, 1).$$

$$(1.45)$$

We may derive asymptotic confidence interval and bounds of [1.9] for $\arcsin\left(\sqrt{\hat{p}_1}\right) - \arcsin\left(\sqrt{\hat{p}_2}\right)$.

[1.9] Asymptotic Confidence Interval and Bounds for Variance-Stabilizing Transformation

The asymptotic confidence interval and bounds for $\arcsin\left(\sqrt{p_1}\right) - \arcsin\left(\sqrt{p_2}\right)$ are expressed by (1)–(3).

(1) The $100(1 - \alpha)\%$ asymptotic confidence interval for $\arcsin\left(\sqrt{p_1}\right) - \arcsin\left(\sqrt{p_2}\right)$ is given by

$$\arcsin\left(\sqrt{p_1}\right) - \arcsin\left(\sqrt{p_2}\right) \in \arcsin\left(\sqrt{\hat{p}_1}\right) - \arcsin\left(\sqrt{\hat{p}_2}\right)$$

$$\pm z(\alpha/2) \cdot \sqrt{\frac{1}{4n_1} + \frac{1}{4n_2}}.$$

(2) The $100(1 - \alpha)\%$ asymptotic lower confidence bound for $\arcsin\left(\sqrt{p_1}\right) - \arcsin\left(\sqrt{p_2}\right)$ is given by

$$\arcsin\left(\sqrt{\hat{p}_1}\right) - \arcsin\left(\sqrt{\hat{p}_2}\right) - z(\alpha) \cdot \sqrt{\frac{1}{4n_1} + \frac{1}{4n_2}}$$

$$< \arcsin\left(\sqrt{p_1}\right) - \arcsin\left(\sqrt{p_2}\right) < \frac{\pi}{2}.$$

(3) The $100(1 - \alpha)\%$ asymptotic upper confidence bound for $\arcsin\left(\sqrt{p_1}\right) - \arcsin\left(\sqrt{p_2}\right)$ is given by

$$-\frac{\pi}{2} < \arcsin\left(\sqrt{p_1}\right) - \arcsin\left(\sqrt{p_2}\right)$$

$$< \arcsin\left(\sqrt{\hat{p}_1}\right) - \arcsin\left(\sqrt{\hat{p}_2}\right) + z(\alpha) \cdot \sqrt{\frac{1}{4n_1} + \frac{1}{4n_2}}.$$

Let us put

$$T_2^s := \frac{2\left\{\arcsin\left(\sqrt{\hat{p}_1}\right) - \arcsin\left(\sqrt{\hat{p}_2}\right)\right\}}{\sqrt{\frac{1}{n_1} + \frac{1}{n_2}}}.$$

Then, from (1.45), we get asymptotic test for the null hypothesis H_0.

[1.10] Asymptotic Tests Based on Variance-Stabilizing Transformation

Whenever $|T_2^s| > z(\alpha/2)$ holds, we reject the null hypothesis H_0 as a test of level α for the null hypothesis H_0 versus the alternative H_1^A.

By the way similar to (1.45), we may derive

$$\frac{\log \hat{p}_1 - \log p_1 - \left(\log \hat{p}_2 + \log p_2\right)}{\sqrt{\frac{1}{n_1 \hat{p}_1} - \frac{1}{n_1} + \frac{1}{n_2 \hat{p}_2} - \frac{1}{n_2}}} \xrightarrow{\mathscr{L}} N(0, 1). \tag{1.46}$$

Hence we may derive asymptotic confidence interval of [1.10] for risk ratio p_1/p_2.

[1.11] Asymptotic Confidence Interval for Risk Ratio

The $100(1 - \alpha)\%$ asymptotic confidence interval for risk ratio p_1/p_2 is given by

$$\frac{p_1}{p_2} \in \frac{\hat{p}_1}{\hat{p}_2} \cdot \exp\left\{\pm z(\alpha/2) \cdot \sqrt{\frac{1}{n_1 \hat{p}_1} - \frac{1}{n_1} + \frac{1}{n_2 \hat{p}_2} - \frac{1}{n_2}}\right\}.$$

Let us put

$$T_2^r := \frac{\log \hat{p}_1 - \log \hat{p}_2}{\sqrt{\frac{1}{n_1 \hat{p}_1} - \frac{1}{n_1} + \frac{1}{n_2 \hat{p}_2} - \frac{1}{n_2}}}.$$

Then, from (1.46), we get asymptotic test for the null hypothesis $H_0^r : p_1/p_2 = 1$.

[1.12] Asymptotic Test for Risk Ratio

Whenever $|T_2^r| > z(\alpha/2)$ holds, we reject the null hypothesis H_0^r as a test of level α for the null hypothesis H_0^r versus the alternative $H_1^{rA} : p_1/p_2 \neq 1$.

By the way similar to (1.45), we may derive

$$\frac{\log\left(\frac{\hat{p}_1}{1-\hat{p}_1}\right) - \log\left(\frac{p_1}{1-p_1}\right) - \left\{\log\left(\frac{\hat{p}_2}{1-\hat{p}_2}\right) - \log\left(\frac{p_2}{1-p_2}\right)\right\}}{\sqrt{\frac{1}{n_1 \hat{p}_1} + \frac{1}{n_1 - n_1 \hat{p}_1} + \frac{1}{n_2 \hat{p}_2} + \frac{1}{n_2 - n_2 \hat{p}_2}}} \xrightarrow{\mathscr{L}} N(0, 1) \tag{1.47}$$

Hence we may derive an asymptotic confidence interval of [1.13] for odds ratio $\frac{\frac{p_1}{1-p_1}}{\frac{p_2}{1-p_2}} = \frac{p_1(1-p_2)}{p_2(1-p_1)}$.

[1.13] Asymptotic Confidence Interval for Odds Ratio

The $100(1 - \alpha)\%$ asymptotic confidence interval for odds ratio $\frac{p_1(1-p_2)}{p_2(1-p_1)}$ is given by

$$\frac{p_1(1 - p_2)}{p_2(1 - p_1)} \in \frac{\hat{p}_1(1 - \hat{p}_2)}{\hat{p}_2(1 - \hat{p}_1)} \cdot \exp\left\{\pm z(\alpha/2) \cdot \hat{q}_n\right\},$$

where

$$\hat{q}_n := \sqrt{\frac{1}{n_1 \hat{p}_1} + \frac{1}{n_1 - n_1 \hat{p}_1} + \frac{1}{n_2 \hat{p}_2} + \frac{1}{n_2 - n_2 \hat{p}_2}}.$$

Let us put

$$T_2^o := \frac{\log\left(\frac{\hat{p}_1}{1-\hat{p}_1}\right) - \log\left(\frac{\hat{p}_2}{1-\hat{p}_2}\right)}{\sqrt{\frac{1}{n_1\hat{p}_1} + \frac{1}{n_1-n_1\hat{p}_1} + \frac{1}{n_2\hat{p}_2} + \frac{1}{n_2-n_2\hat{p}_2}}}.$$

Then, from (1.47), we get asymptotic test for the null hypothesis $H_0^o : \frac{p_1(1-p_2)}{p_2(1-p_1)} = 1$.

[1.14] Asymptotic Test for Odds Ratio

Whenever $|T_2^o| > z(\alpha/2)$ holds, we reject the null hypothesis H_0^o as a test of level α for the null hypothesis H_0^o versus the alternative $H_1^{oA} : \frac{p_1(1-p_2)}{p_2(1-p_1)} \neq 1$.

References

Bickel PJ, Doksum KA (2001) Mathematical statistics Vol 1: Second edition. Prentice Hall
Clopper C, Pearson ES (1934) The use of confidence or fiducial limits illustrated in the case of the binomial. Biometrika 26:404–413
Shiraishi T (2012) An introduction to statistical science. Nippon Hyoron Sha Co Ltd (in Japanese)

Chapter 2
Simultaneous Inference for All Proportions

Abstract We consider multiple comparisons for all proportions in multi-sample models with Bernoulli responses. For binomial models, single-step multiple comparison procedures based on the upper $100\alpha\%$ points of the F-distribution are proposed and discussed. Next closed testing procedures are derived based on the proposed single-step multiple comparison tests. These procedures are exactly conservative. Next the asymptotic theory for the multiple comparisons is discussed. Especially sequentially rejective procedures are constructed in the asymptotic theory.

2.1 Multi-sample Models

We consider k sample models with Bernoulli responses. $(X_{i1}, \ldots, X_{in_i})$ is a random sample of size n_i from the i-th Bernoulli population with success probability p_i $(i = 1, \ldots, k)$. It is convenient to assign the number 1 to a success and the number 0 to a failure.

$$P(X_{ij} = 1) = p_i \text{ and } P(X_{ij} = 0) = 1 - p_i$$

hold. X_{ij}'s are assumed to be independent. The number of successes in the i-th population is given by

$$X_{i\cdot} := X_{i1} + \cdots + X_{in_i}. \tag{2.1}$$

The random variable $X_{i\cdot}$ has a binomial distribution $B(n_i, p_i)$ $(i = 1, \ldots, k)$. The mean and variance of $X_{i\cdot}$ are given by

$$E(X_{i\cdot}) = n_i p_i \text{ and } V(X_{i\cdot}) = n_i p_i (1 - p_i),$$

respectively. Thereafter we assume

$$0 < p_i < 1 \ (i = 1, \ldots, k). \tag{2.2}$$

T. Shiraishi, *Multiple Comparisons for Bernoulli Data*,
JSS Research Series in Statistics,
https://doi.org/10.1007/978-981-19-2708-9_2

2.2 Exact Conservative Procedures

We put

$$\mathscr{I}_k := \{1, \ldots, k\}. \tag{2.3}$$

2.2.1 Single-Step Methods

To construct exact conservative multiple comparison procedures of all p_i's, we impose conditions (c.4) and (c.5).

$$p_i^{n_i} \leq 1 - (1 - \alpha)^{\frac{1}{k}} \quad (i \in \mathscr{I}_k). \tag{c.4}$$

$$(1 - p_i)^{n_i} \leq 1 - (1 - \alpha)^{\frac{1}{k}} \quad (i \in \mathscr{I}_k). \tag{c.5}$$

Theorem 2.1 *For $i \in \mathscr{I}_k$, let us put $K_i := 2(n_i - X_{i\cdot} + 1)$, $L_i := 2X_{i\cdot}$, $K_i^* := 2(X_{i\cdot} + 1)$, and $L_i^* := 2(n_i - X_{i\cdot})$. Then we have the following inequalities (1) and (2).*

(1) Under the condition of (c.4),

$$P\left(\frac{L_i}{K_i \cdot F_{L_i}^{K_i}\left(1 - (1 - \alpha)^{\frac{1}{k}}\right) + L_i} < p_i,\ i \in \mathscr{I}_k \right) \geq 1 - \alpha$$

holds, where $F_{m_2}^{m_1}(\beta)$ is defined in Theorem 1.1.

(2) Under the condition of (c.5),

$$P\left(p_i < \frac{K_i^* \cdot F_{L_i^*}^{K_i^*}\left(1 - (1 - \alpha)^{\frac{1}{k}}\right)}{K_i^* \cdot F_{L_i^*}^{K_i^*}\left(1 - (1 - \alpha)^{\frac{1}{k}}\right) + L_i^*},\ i \in \mathscr{I}_k \right) \geq 1 - \alpha$$

holds.

Proof For $i \in \mathscr{I}_k$, we put

$$G_{1i} := \left\{ \frac{L_i}{K_i \cdot F_{L_i}^{K_i}\left(1 - (1 - \alpha)^{\frac{1}{k}}\right) + L_i} < p_i \right\}.$$

From (1.14), for $i \in \mathscr{I}_k$, we get

$$P\left(G_{1i}\right) \geq (1-\alpha)^{\frac{1}{k}}. \tag{2.4}$$

Since $X_{1.}, \ldots, X_{k.}$ are independent, by using (2.4), we have

$$P\left(\frac{L_i}{K_i \cdot F_{L_i}^{K_i}\left(1-(1-\alpha)^{\frac{1}{k}}\right)+L_i} < p_i, \ i \in \mathscr{I}_k\right) = P\left(\bigcap_{i=1}^{k} G_{1i}\right)$$

$$\geq 1-\alpha.$$

Hence (1) is established. Similarly, by using (1.15), (2) is established. $\quad\square$

We also get Theorem 2.2.

Theorem 2.2 *For $i \in \mathscr{I}_k$, let us put*

$$G_i := \left\{ \frac{L_i}{K_i \cdot F_{L_i}^{K_i}\left(\frac{1-(1-\alpha)^{\frac{1}{k}}}{2}\right)+L_i} < p_i < \frac{K_i^* \cdot F_{L_i^*}^{K_i^*}\left(\frac{1-(1-\alpha)^{\frac{1}{k}}}{2}\right)}{K_i^* \cdot F_{L_i^*}^{K_i^*}\left(\frac{1-(1-\alpha)^{\frac{1}{k}}}{2}\right)+L_i^*} \right\}.$$

Furthermore, add the condition (c.6).

$$p_i^{n_i} \leq \{1-(1-\alpha)^{\frac{1}{k}}\}/2, \quad (1-p_i)^{n_i} \leq \{1-(1-\alpha)^{\frac{1}{k}}\}/2 \quad (i \in \mathscr{I}_k). \tag{c.6}$$

Then

$$P\left(\bigcap_{i=1}^{k} G_i\right) \geq 1-\alpha$$

holds.

Proof From Theorem 1.2, we find

$$P(G_i) \geq (1-\alpha)^{\frac{1}{k}}.$$

Since $G_1, \ldots, G_k$ are independent, we get

$$P\left(\bigcap_{i=1}^{k} G_i\right) = \prod_{i=1}^{k} P(G_i) \geq 1-\alpha,$$

which implies the conclusion. $\quad\square$

From Theorems 2.1 and 2.2, we have confidence intervals and bounds of [2.1].

[2.1] Exact Conservative Confidence Intervals and Bounds for Proportions
The confidence intervals and bounds for $\{p_i |\ i \in \mathscr{I}_k\}$ are expressed by (1)–(3).

(1) Under the condition of (c.6), the $100(1 - \alpha)\%$ simultaneous confidence intervals for $\{p_i \mid i \in \mathscr{I}_k\}$ are given by

$$\frac{L_i}{K_i \cdot F_{L_i}^{K_i}\left(\frac{1-(1-\alpha)^{\frac{1}{k}}}{2}\right) + L_i} < p_i < \frac{K_i^* \cdot F_{L_i^*}^{K_i^*}\left(\frac{1-(1-\alpha)^{\frac{1}{k}}}{2}\right)}{K_i^* \cdot F_{L_i^*}^{K_i^*}\left(\frac{1-(1-\alpha)^{\frac{1}{k}}}{2}\right) + L_i^*} \quad (i \in \mathscr{I}_k).$$

(2) Under the condition (c.4), the $100(1 - \alpha)\%$ simultaneous lower confidence bounds for $\{p_i \mid i \in \mathscr{I}_k\}$ are given by

$$\frac{L_i}{K_i \cdot F_{L_i}^{K_i}\left(1 - (1-\alpha)^{\frac{1}{k}}\right) + L_i} < p_i < 1 \quad (i \in \mathscr{I}_k).$$

(3) Under the condition (c.5), the $100(1 - \alpha)\%$ simultaneous upper confidence bounds for $\{p_i \mid i \in \mathscr{I}_k\}$ are given by

$$0 < p_i < \frac{K_i^* \cdot F_{L_i^*}^{K_i^*}\left(1 - (1-\alpha)^{\frac{1}{k}}\right)}{K_i^* \cdot F_{L_i^*}^{K_i^*}\left(1 - (1-\alpha)^{\frac{1}{k}}\right) + L_i^*} \quad (i \in \mathscr{I}_k).$$

(1) of [2.1] for $k = 1$ is equivalent to (1) of [1.3] given by Clopper and Pearson (1934).

The odds ratio $g(p_i) := p_i/(1 - p_i)$ is strictly increasing in p_i. From [2.1], we have confidence intervals of [2.2] for odds ratios.

[2.2] Exact Conservative Simultaneous Confidence Intervals and Bounds for Odds Ratios

The simultaneous confidence intervals and bounds for $\{p_i/(1 - p_i) \mid i \in \mathscr{I}_k\}$ are expressed by (1)–(3).

(1) Under the condition of (c.6), the $100(1 - \alpha)\%$ simultaneous confidence intervals for $\{p_i/(1 - p_i) \mid i \in \mathscr{I}_k\}$ are given by

$$\frac{L_i}{K_i \cdot F_{L_i}^{K_i}\left(\frac{1-(1-\alpha)^{\frac{1}{k}}}{2}\right)} < \frac{p_i}{1 - p_i} < \frac{K_i^* \cdot F_{L_i^*}^{K_i^*}\left(\frac{1-(1-\alpha)^{\frac{1}{k}}}{2}\right)}{L_i^*} \quad (i \in \mathscr{I}_k).$$

(2) Under the condition (c.4), the $100(1 - \alpha)\%$ simultaneous lower confidence bounds for $\{p_i/(1 - p_i) \mid i \in \mathscr{I}_k\}$ are given by

$$\frac{L_i}{K_i \cdot F_{L_i}^{K_i}\left(1 - (1-\alpha)^{\frac{1}{k}}\right)} < \frac{p_i}{1 - p_i} < 1 \quad (i \in \mathscr{I}_k).$$

(3) Under the condition (c.5), the $100(1 - \alpha)\%$ simultaneous upper confidence bounds for $\{p_i/(1 - p_i) \mid i \in \mathscr{I}_k\}$ are given by

$$0 < \frac{p_i}{1 - p_i} < \frac{K_i^* \cdot F_{L_i^*}^{K_i^*} \left(1 - (1 - \alpha)^{\frac{1}{k}}\right)}{L_i^*} \quad (i \in \mathscr{I}_k).$$

Next, we consider simultaneous tests. We give constants $p_{01}, \ldots, p_{0k}$ such that $0 < p_{01}, \ldots, p_{0k} < 1$. Then we consider three sorts of the following family of hypotheses.

① $\{$the null hypothesis $H_{1i} : p_i = p_{0i}$ vs. the alternative $H_{1i}^A : p_i \neq p_{0i} \mid i \in \mathscr{I}_k\}$

② $\{$the null hypothesis $H_{2i} : p_i \leq p_{0i}$ vs. the alternative $H_{2i}^A : p_i > p_{0i} \mid i \in \mathscr{I}_k\}$

③ $\{$the null hypothesis $H_{3i} : p_i \geq p_{0i}$ vs. the alternative $H_{3i}^A : p_i < p_{0i} \mid i \in \mathscr{I}_k\}.$

From [2.1], we have the test procedures of [2.3].

[2.3] Exact Conservative Simultaneous Tests
The test procedures are given by (1)–(3) for ①–③.

(1) The following condition of (c.7) are added.

$$p_{0i}^{n_i} \leq \{1 - (1 - \alpha)^{\frac{1}{k}}\}/2, \quad (1 - p_{0i})^{n_i} \leq \{1 - (1 - \alpha)^{\frac{1}{k}}\}/2 \quad (i \in \mathscr{I}_k). \quad \text{(c.7)}$$

The simultaneous test of level α for $\{$the null hypothesis H_{1i} vs. the alternative $H_{1i}^A \mid i \in \mathscr{I}_k\}$ consists in rejecting H_{1i} for $i \in \mathscr{I}_k$ such that

$$\frac{L_i}{K_i \cdot F_{L_i}^{K_i} \left(\frac{1 - (1 - \alpha)^{\frac{1}{k}}}{2}\right) + L_i} \geq p_{0i} \text{ or } \frac{K_i^* \cdot F_{L_i^*}^{K_i^*} \left(\frac{1 - (1 - \alpha)^{\frac{1}{k}}}{2}\right)}{K_i^* \cdot F_{L_i^*}^{K_i^*} \left(\frac{1 - (1 - \alpha)^{\frac{1}{k}}}{2}\right) + L_i^*} \leq p_{0i}.$$

(2) Under the condition of

$$p_{0i}^{n_i} \leq 1 - (1 - \alpha)^{\frac{1}{k}} \quad (i \in \mathscr{I}_k),$$

the simultaneous test of level α for $\{$the null hypothesis H_{2i} vs. the alternative $H_{2i}^A \mid i \in \mathscr{I}_k\}$ consists in rejecting H_{2i} for $i \in \mathscr{I}_k$ such that

$$\frac{L_i}{K_i \cdot F_{L_i}^{K_i} \left(1 - (1 - \alpha)^{\frac{1}{k}}\right) + L_i} \geq p_{0i}.$$

(3) Under the condition of

$$(1 - p_{0i})^{n_i} \leq 1 - (1 - \alpha)^{\frac{1}{k}} \quad (i \in \mathscr{I}_k),$$

the simultaneous test of level α for {the null hypothesis H_{3i} vs. the alternative $H_{3i}^A \mid i \in \mathscr{I}_k$} consists in rejecting H_{3i} for $i \in \mathscr{I}_k$ such that

$$\frac{K_i^* \cdot F_{L_i^*}^{K_i^*} \left(1 - (1 - \alpha)^{\frac{1}{k}}\right)}{K_i^* \cdot F_{L_i^*}^{K_i^*} \left(1 - (1 - \alpha)^{\frac{1}{k}}\right) + L_i^*} \leq p_{0i}.$$

2.2.2 Multi-step Methods

Let us put

$$\mathscr{D}_a := \{H_{ai} \mid 1 \leq i \leq k\} = \{H_{ai} \mid i \in \mathscr{I}_k\} \quad (a = 1, 2, 3).$$

Then, the closure of $\mathscr{D}_a$ for any a is given by

$$\overline{\mathscr{D}}_a = \left\{ \bigwedge_{i \in E} H_{ai} \,\middle|\, \emptyset \subsetneq E \subset \mathscr{I}_k \right\}$$

where $\bigwedge$ denotes the conjunction symbol (Refer to Enderton (2001)). Let us define the null hypothesis $H_a(E)$ $(a = 1, 2, 3)$ by

$$H_1(E) : \text{ for any } j \in E, \ p_j = p_{0j} \text{ holds,}$$
$$H_2(E) : \text{ for any } j \in E, \ p_j \leq p_{0j} \text{ holds,}$$
$$H_3(E) : \text{ for any } j \in E, \ p_j \geq p_{0j} \text{ holds.}$$

Then, we get, for $a = 1, 2, 3$,

$$\bigwedge_{i \in E} H_{ai} = H_a(E) \ (\emptyset \subsetneq E \subset \mathscr{I}_k). \tag{2.5}$$

Hence we propose the stepwise procedures [2.4].

[2.4] Stepwise Test Procedures
We give $a \in \{1, 2, 3\}$. Whenever, for any E satisfying $i_0 \in E \subset \mathscr{I}_k$, there exists $j \in E$ such that

$$\begin{cases} \dfrac{L_j}{K_j \cdot F_{L_j}^{K_j}\left(\frac{1-(1-\alpha)^{\frac{1}{\ell}}}{2}\right)+L_j} \geq p_{0j} \text{ or } \dfrac{K_j^* \cdot F_{L_j^*}^{K_j^*}\left(\frac{1-(1-\alpha)^{\frac{1}{\ell}}}{2}\right)}{K_j^* \cdot F_{L_j^*}^{K_j^*}\left(\frac{1-(1-\alpha)^{\frac{1}{\ell}}}{2}\right)+L_j^*} \leq p_{0j} \text{ holds} \\ \qquad\qquad\qquad\qquad\qquad\qquad\qquad\qquad\qquad\qquad\qquad\qquad\qquad\qquad\qquad \text{if } a = 1 \\[2ex] \dfrac{L_j}{K_j \cdot F_{L_j}^{K_j}\left(1-(1-\alpha)^{\frac{1}{\ell}}\right)+L_j} \geq p_{0j} \text{ holds if } a = 2 \\[2ex] \dfrac{K_j^* \cdot F_{L_j^*}^{K_j^*}\left(1-(1-\alpha)^{\frac{1}{\ell}}\right)}{K_j^* \cdot F_{L_j^*}^{K_j^*}\left(1-(1-\alpha)^{\frac{1}{\ell}}\right)+L_j^*} \leq p_{0j} \text{ holds if } a = 3, \end{cases}$$

we reject the null hypothesis H_{ai_0} as a multiple comparison test of level α for {the null hypothesis H_{ai} vs. the alternative $H_{ai}^A \mid i \in \mathscr{I}_k$}, where

$$\ell = \ell(E) := \#(E) \tag{2.6}$$

and $\#(E)$ stands for the number of elements of E.

2.3 Asymptotic Theory

We state asymptotic theory for multiple comparisons. We add the assumption of

$$\lim_{n\to\infty} \frac{n_i}{n} = \lambda_i > 0, \quad (1 \leq i \leq k) \tag{A1}$$

where $n := \sum_{i=1}^k n_i$.

2.3.1 Single-Step Methods

We consider logit transforms

$$\theta_i := \log\left(\frac{p_i}{1-p_i}\right) \text{ and } \hat{\theta}_i := \log\left(\frac{\hat{p}_i}{1-\hat{p}_i}\right),$$

where, by the definition similar to (1.21), $\hat{p}_i$ is given by

$$\hat{p}_i := \frac{X_{i\cdot}}{n_i} \text{ or } \frac{X_{i\cdot}+0.5}{n_i+1}. \tag{2.7}$$

We put, for $\boldsymbol{p} := (p_1, \ldots, p_k)$,

$$T_i(\boldsymbol{p}) := \sqrt{n_i \hat{p}_i(1 - \hat{p}_i)}(\hat{\theta}_i - \theta_i) \text{ or } 2\sqrt{n_i}\left\{\arcsin\left(\sqrt{\hat{p}_i}\right) - \arcsin\left(\sqrt{p_i}\right)\right\}$$

and

$$\widetilde{T}_i(\boldsymbol{p}) := \frac{\sqrt{n_i}(\hat{p}_i - p_i)}{\sqrt{p_i(1 - p_i)}} \text{ or } \frac{\sqrt{n_i}(\hat{p}_i - p_i)}{\sqrt{\hat{p}_i(1 - \hat{p}_i)}}.$$

Theorem 2.3 *Under the condition (A1), for $t > 0$, we have*

$$\lim_{n \to \infty} P\left(\max_{1 \le i \le k} |T_i(\boldsymbol{p})| \le t\right) = \lim_{n \to \infty} P\left(\max_{1 \le i \le k} |\widetilde{T}_i(\boldsymbol{p})| \le t\right) = C_1(t|k), \quad (2.8)$$

and

$$\lim_{n \to \infty} P\left(\max_{1 \le i \le k} T_i(\boldsymbol{p}) \le t\right) = \lim_{n \to \infty} P\left(\max_{1 \le i \le k} \widetilde{T}_i(\boldsymbol{p}) \le t\right) = C_2(t|k), \quad (2.9)$$

where

$$C_1(t|k) := \{2\Phi(t) - 1\}^k \text{ and } C_2(t|k) := \{\Phi(t)\}^k.$$

Proof From (1.22), (1.24), and (1.31), we may derive

$$T_i(\boldsymbol{p}) \xrightarrow{\mathscr{L}} Z_i \sim N(0, 1) \text{ and } \widetilde{T}_i(\boldsymbol{p}) \xrightarrow{\mathscr{L}} Z_i.$$

Since $Z_1, \ldots, Z_k$ are independent, we get

$$\begin{aligned}
\lim_{n \to \infty} P\left(\max_{1 \le i \le k} |T_i(\boldsymbol{p})| \le t\right) &= \lim_{n \to \infty} P\left(\max_{1 \le i \le k} |\widetilde{T}_i(\boldsymbol{p})| \le t\right) \\
&= P\left(\max_{1 \le i \le k} |Z_i| \le t\right) \\
&= \prod_{i=1}^{k} P\left(|Z_i| \le t\right) \\
&= \{\Phi(t) - \Phi(-t)\}^k
\end{aligned}$$

which implies (2.8). Similarly, we get (2.9). □

As a test statistic, let us put

$$T_i := 2\sqrt{n_i}\left\{\arcsin\left(\sqrt{\hat{p}_i}\right) - \arcsin\left(\sqrt{p_{0i}}\right)\right\} \text{ or } \frac{\sqrt{n_i}(\hat{p}_i - p_{0i})}{\sqrt{\hat{p}_i(1 - \hat{p}_i)}}. \quad (2.10)$$

Then, from Theorem 2.3, we get Corollary 2.1.

Corollary 2.1 *Under (A1), for $t > 0$, we have*

$$\lim_{n\to\infty} P_0\left(\max_{1\le i\le k} |T_i| \le t\right) = C_1(t|k) \quad and \quad \lim_{n\to\infty} P_0\left(\max_{1\le i\le k} T_i \le t\right) = C_2(t|k),$$

where $P_0(\cdot)$ denotes the probability measure under the condition of $p_i = p_{0i}$ ($1 \le i \le k$). □

For a given α such that $0 < \alpha < 1$, we put

$$c_1(k; \alpha) := \text{a solution of } t \text{ satisfying the equation } C_1(t|k) = 1 - \alpha \quad (2.11)$$

and

$$c_2(k; \alpha) := \text{a solution of } t \text{ satisfying the equation } C_2(t|k) = 1 - \alpha. \quad (2.12)$$

From Corollary 2.1, we have the test procedures of [2.5].

[2.5] Asymptotic Simultaneous Tests
The test procedures are given by (1)–(3).

(1) The asymptotic simultaneous test of level α for {the null hypothesis H_{1i} vs. the alternative $H_{1i}^A \mid i \in \mathscr{I}_k$} consists in rejecting H_{1i} for $i \in \mathscr{I}_k$ such that $|T_i| > c_1(k; \alpha)$.

(2) The asymptotic simultaneous test of level α for {the null hypothesis H_{2i} vs. the alternative $H_{2i}^A \mid i \in \mathscr{I}_k$} consists in rejecting H_{2i} for $i \in \mathscr{I}_k$ such that $T_i > c_2(k; \alpha)$.

(3) The asymptotic simultaneous test of level α for {the null hypothesis H_{3i} vs. the alternative $H_{3i}^A \mid i \in \mathscr{I}_k$} consists in rejecting H_{3i} for $i \in \mathscr{I}_k$ such that $-T_i > c_2(k; \alpha)$.

Let us put

$$U_i := 1/\sqrt{n_i \hat{p}_i(1 - \hat{p}_i)} \ (i \in \mathscr{I}_k).$$

Then, from Theorem 2.3, the $100(1 - \alpha)\%$ asymptotic simultaneous confidence intervals for $\{\theta_i \mid i \in \mathscr{I}_k\}$ are given by

$$\hat{\theta}_i - c_1(k; \alpha) \cdot U_i < \theta_i < \hat{\theta}_i + c_1(k; \alpha) \cdot U_i \ (i \in \mathscr{I}_k). \quad (2.13)$$

From (2.13) and (1.29), the $100(1 - \alpha)\%$ asymptotic simultaneous confidence intervals for $\{p_i \mid i \in \mathscr{I}_k\}$ are given by

$$\frac{\exp\left\{\hat{\theta}_i - c_1(k; \alpha) \cdot U_i\right\}}{1 + \exp\left\{\hat{\theta}_i - c_1(k; \alpha) \cdot U_i\right\}} < p_i < \frac{\exp\left\{\hat{\theta}_i + c_1(k; \alpha) \cdot U_i\right\}}{1 + \exp\left\{\hat{\theta}_i + c_1(k; \alpha) \cdot U_i\right\}} \ (i \in \mathscr{I}_k).$$

These intervals do not include 0 and 1. On the other hand, although

$$\hat{p}_i - c_1(k;\alpha) \cdot \sqrt{\frac{\hat{p}_i(1-\hat{p}_i)}{n_i}} < p_i < \hat{p}_i + c_1(k;\alpha) \cdot \sqrt{\frac{\hat{p}_i(1-\hat{p}_i)}{n_i}} \quad (i \in \mathscr{I}_k)$$

and

$$\frac{2n_i\hat{p}_i + \{c_1(k;\alpha)\}^2 - \sqrt{4n_i\{c_1(k;\alpha)\}^2\hat{p}_i(1-\hat{p}_i) + \{c_1(k;\alpha)\}^4}}{2(n_i + \{c_1(k;\alpha)\}^2)}$$

$$< p_i < \frac{2n_i\hat{p}_i + \{c_1(k;\alpha)\}^2 + \sqrt{4n_i\{c_1(k;\alpha)\}^2\hat{p}_i(1-\hat{p}_i) + \{c_1(k;\alpha)\}^4}}{2(n_i + \{c_1(k;\alpha)\}^2)} \quad (i \in \mathscr{I}_k)$$

are $100(1-\alpha)\%$ asymptotic simultaneous confidence intervals for $\{p_i \mid i \in \mathscr{I}_k\}$, these intervals may include 0 or 1. Similarly asymptotic simultaneous one-sided confidence intervals are derived. We summarize these procedures.

[2.6] Asymptotic Simultaneous Confidence Intervals
The simultaneous confidence intervals and bounds for $\{p_i \mid i \in \mathscr{I}_k\}$ are expressed by (1)–(3).

(1) Under the condition of (A1), the $100(1-\alpha)\%$ simultaneous confidence intervals for $\{p_i \mid i \in \mathscr{I}_k\}$ are given by

$$\frac{\exp\left\{\hat{\theta}_i - c_1(k;\alpha) \cdot U_i\right\}}{1 + \exp\left\{\hat{\theta}_i - c_1(k;\alpha) \cdot U_i\right\}} < p_i < \frac{\exp\left\{\hat{\theta}_i + c_1(k;\alpha) \cdot U_i\right\}}{1 + \exp\left\{\hat{\theta}_i + c_1(k;\alpha) \cdot U_i\right\}} \quad (i \in \mathscr{I}_k)$$

and

$$\sin^2\left[\max\left\{\arcsin\left(\sqrt{\hat{p}_i}\right) - \frac{c_1(k;\alpha)}{2\sqrt{n_i}}, \, 0\right\}\right]$$

$$< p < \sin^2\left[\min\left\{\arcsin\left(\sqrt{\hat{p}_i}\right) + \frac{c_1(k;\alpha)}{2\sqrt{n_i}}, \, \frac{\pi}{2}\right\}\right] \quad (i \in \mathscr{I}_k).$$

(2) Under the condition of (A1), the $100(1-\alpha)\%$ simultaneous confidence lower bounds for $\{p_i \mid i \in \mathscr{I}_k\}$ are given by

$$\frac{\exp\left\{\hat{\theta}_i - c_2(k;\alpha) \cdot U_i\right\}}{1 + \exp\left\{\hat{\theta}_i - c_2(k;\alpha) \cdot U_i\right\}} < p_i < 1 \quad (i \in \mathscr{I}_k).$$

(3) Under the condition of (A1), the $100(1-\alpha)\%$ simultaneous confidence upper bounds for $\{p_i \mid i \in \mathscr{I}_k\}$ are given by

$$0 < p_i < \frac{\exp\left\{\hat{\theta}_i + c_2(k; \alpha) \cdot U_i\right\}}{1 + \exp\left\{\hat{\theta}_i + c_2(k; \alpha) \cdot U_i\right\}} \quad (i \in \mathscr{I}_k).$$

2.3.2 Sequentially Rejective Multiple Test Procedures

For $a = 1, 2, 3$ in (2.5), we define the statistic T_i^* $(i \in \mathscr{I}_k)$ by

$$T_i^* := \begin{cases} |T_i| & (a = 1) \\ T_i & (a = 2) \\ -T_i & (a = 3). \end{cases}$$

We put, for $\ell = 1, \ldots, k$,

$$c^*(\ell; \alpha) := \begin{cases} c_1(\ell; \alpha) & (a = 1) \\ c_2(\ell; \alpha) & (a = 2) \\ c_2(\ell; \alpha) & (a = 3), \end{cases}$$

where $c_1(\ell; \alpha)$ and $c_2(\ell; \alpha)$ are given by replacing k with ℓ in (2.11) and (2.12), respectively. Whenever, for any E $(\subset \mathscr{I}_k)$ such that $i_0 \in E$, $\max_{i \in E} T_i^* > c^*(\ell; \alpha)$ holds, we may reject the null hypothesis H_{ai_0} as a multiple comparison test of level α for {the null hypothesis H_{ai} vs. the alternative $H_{ai}^A \mid i \in \mathscr{I}_k$}, where E and $H_a(E)$ appear in (2.5) and $\ell := \#(E)$.

Let $T_{(1)}^* \leq T_{(2)}^* \leq \cdots \leq T_{(k)}^*$ be the ordered statistics of T_i^*'s and let $H_{a(1)}, \ldots, H_{a(k)}$ be the corresponding hypotheses. Then we get multi-step procedures [2.7].

[2.7] Sequentially Rejective Test Procedures

We give $a \in \{1, 2, 3\}$. For ℓ such that $1 \leq \ell \leq k$, we proceed as follows.

(Step 1) We put $\ell = k$.

(Step 2)

(i) If $T_{(\ell)}^* \leq c^*(\ell; \alpha)$, $H_{a(1)}, \ldots, H_{a(\ell)}$ are not rejected. Finish this test procedure.

(ii) If $T_{(\ell)}^* > c^*(\ell; \alpha)$, $H_{a(\ell)}$ is rejected and go to step 3.

(Step 3)

(i) When $\ell \geq 2$, set $\ell - 1$ as ℓ and return step 2.

(ii) When $\ell = 2$, finish this test procedure.

The test procedures [2.7] are asymptotically multiple comparison tests of level α.

References

Clopper C, Pearson ES (1934) The use of confidence or fiducial limits illustrated in the case of the binomial. Biometrika 26:404–413

Enderton HB (2001) A mathematical introduction to logic, 2nd edn. Academic, New York

Chapter 3
All-Pairwise Comparison Tests

Abstract We consider multiple tests for the differences among proportions in k binomial populations. The simultaneous confidence intervals for all the pairwise differences among the proportions are expressed in Hochberg and Tamhane (1987). We may propose the Tukey-Kramer type multiple tests similar to the simultaneous confidence intervals. However, the degree of the conservativeness for the multiple tests depends on unknown parameters. Therefore multiple tests based on arcsine transformation are proposed. It is shown that the degree of the conservativeness for the proposed tests is controlled by the sizes of the samples.

3.1 Introduction

We consider k sample models with Bernoulli responses. $(X_{i1}, \ldots, X_{in_i})$ is a random sample of size n_i from the i-th Bernoulli population with success probability p_i $(i = 1, \ldots, k)$. It is convenient to assign the number 1 to a success and the number 0 to a failure. The settings for this model are same as in Sect. 2.1.

We consider testing the null hypothesis of homogeneity

$$H_0 : \ p_1 = \ldots = p_k. \tag{3.1}$$

Let us put

$$S := 4 \sum_{i=1}^{k} n_i \left\{ \arcsin\left(\sqrt{\hat{p}_i}\right) - \sum_{j=1}^{k} \left(\frac{n_j}{n}\right) \arcsin\left(\sqrt{\hat{p}_j}\right) \right\}^2 \tag{3.2}$$

and add the assumption of

© The Author(s), under exclusive license to Springer Nature Singapore Pte Ltd. 2022
T. Shiraishi, *Multiple Comparisons for Bernoulli Data*,
JSS Research Series in Statistics,
https://doi.org/10.1007/978-981-19-2708-9_3

$$(A1) \qquad\qquad\qquad \lim_{n \to \infty} \frac{n_i}{n} = \lambda_i > 0, \quad (1 \le i \le k)$$

where $n := \sum_{i=1}^{k} n_i$. Then Shiraishi and Matsuda (2016) showed that, under H_0 and under the assumption of (A1), as $n \to \infty$, S has asymptotic χ^2-distribution with $k-1$ degrees of freedom. Hence we reject H_0 at level α for the null hypothesis if $S > \chi_{k-1}^2(\alpha)$, where $\chi_{k-1}^2(\alpha)$ denotes the upper $100\alpha\%$ point of χ^2-distribution with $k-1$ degrees of freedom. For specified i, i' such that $1 \le i < i' \le k$, if we are interested in testing

the null hypothesis $H_{(i,i')} : p_i = p_{i'}$ versus the alternative $H_{(i,i')}^A : p_i \ne p_{i'}$, (3.3)

we can use the two-sided two-sample z-test. In this chapter, we consider test procedures for all-pairwise comparisons of $\{$the null hypothesis $H_{(i,i')}$ versus the alternative $H_{(i,i')}^A \big| (i, i') \in \mathcal{U}_k \}$, where

$$\mathcal{U}_k = \{(i, i') \mid 1 \le i < i' \le k\}. \tag{3.4}$$

Tukey (1953) and Kramer (1956) proposed single-step procedures as multiple comparison tests of level α in homoscedastic k sample model under normality. Shiraishi (2011a) proposed closed testing procedures. Shiraishi (2011b) and Shiraishi, et al. (2019) show that (i) the proposed multi-step procedures are more powerful than single-step procedures and the REGW (Ryan–Einot–Gabriel–Welsch) tests, and (ii) confidence regions induced by the multi-step procedures are equivalent to simultaneous confidence intervals. The REGW test procedures are included in the SPSS system.

Procedures and theory stated in this chapter are used in hybrid serial gatekeeping procedures for all-pairwise comparisons of Chap. 8.

3.2 Single-Step Test Procedures

The estimator $\hat{p}_i$ for p_i is given by

$$\hat{p}_i := \frac{X_{i\cdot}}{n_i} \quad \text{or} \quad \frac{X_{i\cdot} + 0.5}{n_i + 1}, \tag{3.5}$$

where $X_{i\cdot} := \sum_{j=1}^{n_i} X_{ij}$. We put, for $(i, i') \in \mathcal{U}_k$,

$$T_{i'i}(\boldsymbol{p}) := \frac{2\left\{\arcsin\left(\sqrt{\hat{p}_{i'}}\right) - \arcsin\left(\sqrt{\hat{p}_i}\right) - \arcsin\left(\sqrt{p_{i'}}\right) + \arcsin\left(\sqrt{p_i}\right)\right\}}{\sqrt{\frac{1}{n_i} + \frac{1}{n_{i'}}}},$$

(3.6)

$$T_{i'i} := \frac{2\left\{\arcsin\left(\sqrt{\hat{p}_{i'}}\right) - \arcsin\left(\sqrt{\hat{p}_i}\right)\right\}}{\sqrt{\frac{1}{n_i} + \frac{1}{n_{i'}}}},$$

(3.7)

$$\widetilde{T}_{i'i}(\boldsymbol{p}) := \frac{\hat{p}_{i'} - \hat{p}_i - p_{i'} + p_i}{\sqrt{\frac{1}{n_i}\hat{p}_i(1 - \hat{p}_i) + \frac{1}{n_{i'}}\hat{p}_{i'}(1 - \hat{p}_{i'})}},$$

(3.8)

$$\widetilde{T}_{i'i} := \frac{\hat{p}_{i'} - \hat{p}_i}{\sqrt{\frac{1}{n_i}\hat{p}_i(1 - \hat{p}_i) + \frac{1}{n_{i'}}\hat{p}_{i'}(1 - \hat{p}_{i'})}},$$

(3.9)

where $\boldsymbol{p} := (p_1, \ldots, p_k)$.

We state asymptotic theory for multiple comparisons. From (1.22) and (1.24), under the assumption of (A1), as $n \to \infty$, we have

$$\sqrt{n}(\hat{p}_i - p_i) \overset{\mathscr{L}}{\to} Y_i \sim N\left(0, \frac{p_i(1 - p_i)}{\lambda_i}\right)$$

(3.10)

and

$$2\sqrt{n}\left\{\arcsin\left(\sqrt{\hat{p}_i}\right) - \arcsin\left(\sqrt{p_i}\right)\right\} \overset{\mathscr{L}}{\to} Z_i \sim N\left(0, \frac{1}{\lambda_i}\right).$$

(3.11)

By using (3.10) and (3.11), we get Theorem 3.1.

Theorem 3.1 *For $t > 0$, under the assumption of (A1), we have*

$$A(t|k) \le \lim_{n\to\infty} P\left(\max_{1\le i < i' \le k} |T_{i'i}(\boldsymbol{p})| \le t\right) \le A^*(t|k, \boldsymbol{\lambda}),$$

(3.12)

$$\lim_{n\to\infty} P\left(\max_{1\le i < i' \le k} |T_{i'i}(\boldsymbol{p})| \le t\right) = \lim_{n\to\infty} P_0\left(\max_{1\le i < i' \le k} |T_{i'i}| \le t\right),$$

(3.13)

$$A(t|k) \le \lim_{n\to\infty} P\left(\max_{1\le i < i' \le k} |\widetilde{T}_{i'i}(\boldsymbol{p})| \le t\right) \le A^*(t|k, \boldsymbol{q}),$$

(3.14)

$$\lim_{n\to\infty} P\left(\max_{1\le i < i' \le k} |\widetilde{T}_{i'i}(\boldsymbol{p})| \le t\right) \ne \lim_{n\to\infty} P_0\left(\max_{1\le i < i' \le k} |\widetilde{T}_{i'i}| \le t\right),$$

(3.15)

where $P_0(\cdot)$ stands for the probability measure under the null hypothesis H_0,

Table 3.1 The values of $a(k; \alpha)$ for the single-step procedures [3.1] and [3.2]

$100\alpha\%$ \ k	2	3	4	5	6	7	8	9	10
5%	1.960	2.344	2.569	2.728	2.850	2.948	3.031	3.102	3.164
1%	2.576	2.913	3.113	3.255	3.364	3.452	3.526	3.590	3.646

$$A(t|k) := k \int_{-\infty}^{\infty} \{\Phi(x) - \Phi(x - \sqrt{2} \cdot t)\}^{k-1} d\Phi(x), \tag{3.16}$$

$$A^*(t|k, \boldsymbol{\lambda}) := \int_{-\infty}^{\infty} \sum_{j=1}^{k} \prod_{\substack{i=1 \\ i \neq j}}^{k} \left\{ \Phi\left(\sqrt{\frac{\lambda_i}{\lambda_j}} \cdot x\right) - \Phi\left(\sqrt{\frac{\lambda_i}{\lambda_j}} \cdot x - \sqrt{\frac{\lambda_i + \lambda_j}{\lambda_j}} \cdot t\right) \right\} d\Phi(x),$$

$$A^*(t|k, \boldsymbol{q}) := \int_{-\infty}^{\infty} \sum_{j=1}^{k} \prod_{\substack{i=1 \\ i \neq j}}^{k} \left\{ \Phi\left(\sqrt{\frac{q_j}{q_i}} \cdot x\right) - \Phi\left(\sqrt{\frac{q_j}{q_i}} \cdot x - \sqrt{\frac{q_j + q_i}{q_i}} \cdot t\right) \right\} d\Phi(x),$$

$$\tag{3.17}$$

$$\boldsymbol{\lambda} := (\lambda_1, \ldots, \lambda_k), \ \boldsymbol{q} := (q_1, \ldots, q_k), \tag{3.18}$$

and

$$q_i := p_i(1 - p_i)/\lambda_i \ (i = 1, \ldots, k). \tag{3.19}$$

When $\lambda_1 = \ldots = \lambda_k$ is satisfied, the both inequalities of (3.12) become equalities.
□

The left-hand side of the inequalities in (3.12) is derived from main theorem of Hayter (1984). The right-hand side of the inequalities in (3.12) is given by Shiraishi (2006). The two inequalities of (3.14) are also proved similarly. For a given α such that $0 < \alpha < 1$, we put

$$a(k; \alpha) := (\text{a solution of } t \text{ satisfying the equation } A(t|k) = 1 - \alpha). \tag{3.20}$$

For $\alpha = 0.05, \ 0.01$, we give the values of $a(k; \alpha)$ in Table 3.1. We limited attention to $2 \leq k \leq 10$.

From the left-hand side of the inequality (3.12), we get asymptotic simultaneous test of [3.1].

[3.1] Tukey-Kramer Type Test Based on Arcsine Transformation
The Tukey-Kramer type test of level α for {the null hypothesis $H_{(i,i')}$ versus the alternative $H_{(i,i')}^{A}| \ (i, i') \in \mathscr{U}_k$} consists in rejecting $H_{(i,i')}$ for $(i, i') \in \mathscr{U}_k$ such that $|T_{i'i}| > a(k; \alpha)$.

We put

$$\Theta_0 := \{\boldsymbol{p} \mid \text{at least one null hypothesis } H_{(i,i')} \text{ is true}\}$$
$$= \{\boldsymbol{p} \mid \text{there exists } (i, i') \in \mathcal{U}_k \text{ such that } p_i = p_{i'}\}. \tag{3.21}$$

We take $\boldsymbol{p}_0 := (p_{01}, \cdots, p_{0k}) \in \Theta_0$. Suppose $\boldsymbol{p} = \boldsymbol{p}_0$. Then we decide the set $\mathcal{A}(\boldsymbol{p}_0)$ such that $H_{(i,i')}$ is true $(p_{0i} = p_{0i'})$ for any $(i, i') \in \mathcal{A}(\boldsymbol{p}_0) \subset \mathcal{U}_k$ and $H_{(i,i')}$ is false $(p_{0i} \neq p_{0i'})$ for any $(i, i') \in \{\mathcal{A}(\boldsymbol{p}_0)\}^c \cap \mathcal{U}_k$. $\mathcal{A}(\boldsymbol{p}_0) \neq \emptyset$ holds. $\{H_{(i,i')} \mid (i, i') \in \mathcal{A}(\boldsymbol{p}_0)\}$ is a family of true null hypotheses. From the left-hand side of the inequality (3.12), the probability of rejecting at least one true null hypothesis is given by

$$\lim_{n \to \infty} P_{\boldsymbol{p}_0} \left(\max_{(i,i') \in \mathcal{A}(\boldsymbol{p}_0)} |T_{i'i}| > a(k; \alpha) \right) = \lim_{n \to \infty} P_{\boldsymbol{p}_0} \left(\max_{(i,i') \in \mathcal{A}(\boldsymbol{p}_0)} |T_{i'i}(p_0)| > a(k; \alpha) \right)$$

$$\leq \lim_{n \to \infty} P_{\boldsymbol{p}_0} \left(\max_{(i,i') \in \mathcal{U}_k} |T_{i'i}(p_0)| > a(k; \alpha) \right)$$

$$= \lim_{n \to \infty} P_0 \left(\max_{(i,i') \in \mathcal{U}_k} |T_{i'i}| > a(k; \alpha) \right)$$

$$\leq 1 - A(a(k; \alpha)|k)$$

$$= \alpha, \tag{3.22}$$

where $P_{\boldsymbol{p}_0}(\cdot)$ denotes the probability measure under $\boldsymbol{p} = \boldsymbol{p}_0$.

From the left-hand side of the inequality (3.14), we get asymptotic simultaneous test of [3.2].

[3.2] Simple Single-Step Test

The simple Tukey-Kramer type test of level α for {the null hypothesis $H_{(i,i')}$ versus the alternative $H_{(i,i')}^A \mid (i, i') \in \mathcal{U}_k\}$ consists in rejecting $H_{(i,i')}$ for $(i, i') \in \mathcal{U}_k$ such that $|\widetilde{T}_{i'i}| > a(k; \alpha)$.

From the left inequality of (3.12), we find that the Tukey-Kramer type test of [3.1] is conservative. Under the condition of $\max_{1 \leq i \leq k} \lambda_i / \min_{1 \leq i \leq k} \lambda_i \leq 2$, Shiraishi (2006) found that the values of $A^*(t|k, \boldsymbol{\lambda}) - A(t|k)$ is nearly equal to 0 for various values of t from numerical integration. Therefore the conservativeness of the Tukey-Kramer type method [3.1] is small. On the other hand, $\lim_{n \to \infty} P \left(\max_{(i,i') \in \mathcal{U}_k} |\widetilde{T}_{i'i}(\boldsymbol{p})| \leq t \right)$ depends on unknown parameters $p_1, \ldots, p_k$. Therefore (3.14) may not control the conservativeness of [3.2]. Hence simultaneous test of [3.1] is preferable to [3.2].

3.3 Closed Testing Procedures

Let us put

$$\mathcal{H}_1 := \{H_{(i,i')} \mid (i, i') \in \mathcal{U}_k\}. \tag{3.23}$$

Then, the closure of $\mathcal{H}_1$ is given by

$$\overline{\mathcal{H}_1} = \left\{ \bigwedge_{v \in V} H_v \mid \emptyset \subsetneq V \subset \mathcal{U}_k \right\},$$

where $\bigwedge$ denotes the conjunction symbol (Refer to Enderton (2001)). Then, we get

$$\bigwedge_{v \in V} H_v : \text{for any } (i, i') \in V, \ p_i = p_{i'} \text{ holds.} \tag{3.24}$$

For an integer J and disjoint sets $I_1, \ldots, I_J \subset \{1, \ldots, k\}$, we define the null hypothesis $H(I_1, \ldots, I_J)$ by

$$H(I_1, \ldots, I_J) : \text{for any integer } j \text{ such that } 1 \leq j \leq J$$
$$\text{and for any } i, i' \in I_j, \ p_i = p_{i'} \text{ holds.} \tag{3.25}$$

From (3.24) and (3.25), for any nonempty $V \subset \mathcal{U}_k$, there exist an integer J and disjoint sets $I_1, \ldots, I_J$ such that

$$\bigwedge_{v \in V} H_v = H(I_1, \ldots, I_J) \tag{3.26}$$

and $\#(I_j) \geq 2 \ (j = 1, \ldots, J)$, where $\#(A)$ stands for the cardinal number of set A. For $H(I_1, \ldots, I_J)$ of (3.26), we set

$$M := M(I_1, \ldots, I_J) := \sum_{j=1}^{J} \ell_j, \ \ell_j := \#(I_j). \tag{3.27}$$

Let us put

$$T(I_j) := \max_{i < i', \ i, i' \in I_j} |T_{i'i}| \quad (j = 1, \ldots, J).$$

Then, we propose the stepwise procedure [3.3].

[3.3] Stepwise Procedure Based on Arcsine Transformation
For $\ell = \ell_1, \ldots, \ell_J$, we define $\alpha(M, \ell)$ by

$$\alpha(M, \ell) := 1 - (1 - \alpha)^{\ell/M}. \tag{3.28}$$

Corresponding to (3.12), we put

$$A(t|\ell) := \ell \int_{-\infty}^{\infty} \{\Phi(x) - \Phi(x - \sqrt{2} \cdot t)\}^{\ell-1} d\Phi(x). \tag{3.29}$$

Table 3.2 The values of $a(\ell; \alpha(M, \ell))$ for the stepwise procedure [3.3] with $\alpha = 0.05$

$M \setminus \ell$	2	3	4	5	6	7	8	9	10
10	2.569	2.774	2.887	2.964	3.021	3.066	3.104	◊	3.164
9	2.532	2.739	2.852	2.929	2.986	3.032	◊	3.102	
8	2.491	2.699	2.813	2.890	2.947	◊	3.031		
7	2.443	2.653	2.767	2.845	◊	2.948			
6	2.388	2.599	2.714	◊	2.850				
5	2.321	2.534	◊	2.728					
4	2.236	◊	2.569						
3	◊	2.344							
2	1.960								

The places of ◊ are not used in the procedure [3.3]

By obeying the notation $a(k; \alpha)$, we get

$$A(a(\ell; \alpha(M, \ell))|\ell) = 1 - \alpha(M, \ell) = (1 - \alpha)^{\ell/M}, \qquad (3.30)$$

that is, $a(\ell; \alpha(M, \ell))$ is an upper $100\alpha(M, \ell)\%$ point of the distribution $A(t|\ell)$.

(a) $J \geq 2$

Whenever $a\left(\ell_j; \alpha(M, \ell_j)\right) < T(I_j)$ holds for an integer j such that $1 \leq j \leq J$, we reject the hypothesis $\bigwedge_{v \in V} H_v$.

(b) $J = 1$ $(M = \ell_1)$

Whenever $a(M; \alpha) < T(I_1)$ holds, we reject the hypothesis $\bigwedge_{v \in V} H_v$.

By using the methods of (a) and (b), when $\bigwedge_{v \in V} H_v$ is rejected for any V such that $(i, i') \in V \subset \mathcal{U}_k$, the null hypothesis $H_{(i,i')}$ is rejected as a multiple comparison test.

For $\alpha = 0.05$, 0.01, we give the values of $a(\ell; \alpha(M, \ell))$ in Tables 3.2 and 3.3, respectively. We limited attention to $2 \leq M \leq 10$. $\ell = M - 1$ is not used in the procedure [3.3]. When $\ell = M = k$ is satisfied, $a(\ell; \alpha(M, \ell)) = a(k; \alpha)$ holds.

Theorem 3.2 *Under the assumption of (A1), as $n \to \infty$, the test procedure [3.3] is an asymptotic multiple comparison test of level α.*

Proof It is trivial to verify that the asymptotic level of the test procedure of (b) is α. We show that the asymptotic level of the test procedure of (a) is α. Furthermore, we suppose without any loss of generality that H_0 is true. Since $T(I_1), \ldots, T(I_J)$ are independent, we get

$$\lim_{n \to \infty} P_0\left(T(I_j) \leq a\left(\ell_j; \alpha(M, \ell_j)\right), \; j = 1, \ldots, J\right)$$

$$= \prod_{j=1}^{J}\left\{\lim_{n \to \infty} P_0\left(T(I_j) \leq a\left(\ell_j; \alpha(M, \ell_j)\right)\right)\right\}. \qquad (3.31)$$

Table 3.3 The values of $a(\ell; \alpha(M, \ell))$ for the stepwise procedure [3.3] with $\alpha = 0.01$

$M \setminus \ell$	2	3	4	5	6	7	8	9	10
10	3.089	3.277	3.382	3.454	3.508	3.552	3.588	$\Diamond$	3.646
9	3.058	3.247	3.352	3.424	3.479	3.523	$\Diamond$	3.590	
8	3.022	3.213	3.318	3.391	3.446	$\Diamond$	3.526		
7	2.982	3.173	3.280	3.353	$\Diamond$	3.452			
6	2.934	3.128	3.235	$\Diamond$	3.364				
5	2.877	3.073	$\Diamond$	3.255					
4	2.806	$\Diamond$	3.113						
3	$\Diamond$	2.913							
2	2.576								

From the left-hand side of the inequality (3.12), we have

$$(3.31) \geq \prod_{j=1}^{J} A\left(a(\ell_j; \alpha(M, \ell_j))\big|\ell_j\right)$$

$$= \prod_{j=1}^{J} \left(1 - \alpha(M, \ell_j)\right)$$

$$= \prod_{j=1}^{J} \left\{(1 - \alpha)^{\ell_j/M}\right\}$$

$$= 1 - \alpha. \tag{3.32}$$

By using (3.32), we get

$$\lim_{n \to \infty} P_0\left(\text{There exists } j \text{ such that } T(I_j) > a\left(\ell_j; \alpha(M, \ell_j)\right)\right)$$

$$= 1 - \lim_{n \to \infty} P_0\left(T(I_j) \leq a\left(\ell_j; \alpha(M, \ell_j)\right), \ j = 1, \ldots, J\right)$$

$$\leq 1 - \prod_{j=1}^{J} \left\{(1 - \alpha)^{\ell_j/M}\right\}$$

$$= \alpha. \tag{3.33}$$

Therefore, the level of the test procedure of (a) for the null hypothesis $\bigwedge_{v \in V} H_v$ is α. $\qquad\square$

From (3.26), we find

$$\overline{\mathcal{H}_1} = \{H(I_1, \ldots, I_J) \mid \text{There exists } J \text{ such that}$$

$$\bigcup_{j=1}^{J} I_j \subset \{1, \ldots, k\}, \ \#(I_j) \geq 2 \ (1 \leq j \leq J),$$

$$\text{and } I_j \cap I_{j'} = \emptyset \ (1 \leq j < j' \leq J) \text{ are satisfied if } J \geq 2.\}$$

For $(i, i') \in \mathcal{U}_k$, let us put

$$\overline{\mathcal{H}_1}_{(i,i')} := \{H(I_1, \ldots, I_J) \in \overline{\mathcal{H}_1} \mid \text{There exists } j \text{ such that } \{i, i'\} \subset I_j \text{ and } 1 \leq j \leq J\}.$$

Then we get

$$\overline{\mathcal{H}_1} = \bigcup_{(i,i') \in \mathcal{U}_k} \overline{\mathcal{H}_1}_{(i,i')} \quad \text{and} \quad H_{(i,i')}, \ H_0 \in \overline{\mathcal{H}_1}_{(i,i')}.$$

Therefore, by following (i) and (ii), we make a decision to reject or retain $H_{(i,i')}$ as a multiple comparison test of level α for $(i, i') \in \mathcal{U}_k$.

(i) Whenever all the elements of $\overline{\mathcal{H}_1}_{(i,i')}$ are rejected, $H_{(i,i')}$ is rejected.
(ii) Whenever there exists an element of $\overline{\mathcal{H}_1}_{(i,i')}$ that is not rejected, $H_{(i,i')}$ is not rejected.

For $k = 4$, all the elements $H(I_1, \ldots, I_J)$ of $\overline{\mathcal{H}_1}_{(1,2)}$ are stated in Table 3.4. From Table 3.4, in order to reject $H_{(1,2)}$ as a multiple comparison test, five null hypotheses must be rejected. Whenever the following (3-1)–(3-5) are satisfied, the closed testing procedure of [3.3] rejects $H_{(1,2)}$ as a multiple comparison test of level 0.05.

(3-1) $T(\{1, 2, 3, 4\}) = \max_{1 \leq i < i' \leq 4} |T_{i'i}| > a(4; \alpha) = 2.569$
(3-2) $T(\{1, 2\}) = |T_{21}| > a(2; \alpha(4, 2)) = 2.236$ or $T(\{3, 4\}) = |T_{43}| > a(2; \alpha(4, 2)) = 2.236$
(3-3) $T(\{1, 2, 3\}) = \max_{1 \leq i < i' \leq 3} |T_{i'i}| > a(3; \alpha) = 2.344$
(3-4) $T(\{1, 2, 4\}) = \max\{|T_{21}|, |T_{41}|, |T_{42}|\} > a(3; \alpha) = 2.344$
(3-5) $T(\{1, 2\}) = |T_{21}| > a(2; \alpha) = 1.960$

For $k = 5$, all the elements $H(I_1, \ldots, I_J)$ of $\overline{\mathcal{H}_1}_{(1,2)}$ are stated in Table 3.5.

From a definition, we can verify that $a(\ell; \alpha) < a(k; \alpha)$ holds for ℓ such that $2 \leq \ell < k$. For $\alpha = 0.05, 0.01$, we give the values of $a(\ell; \alpha(M, \ell))$ in Tables 3.2 and 3.3, respectively. We limited attention to $2 \leq M \leq 10$. $\ell = M - 1$ is not used in the procedure [3.3]. When $\ell = M = k$ is satisfied, $a(\ell; \alpha(M, \ell)) = a(k; \alpha)$ holds.

For $\alpha = 0.05, 0.01$, and $4 \leq k \leq 10$, from Tables 3.2 and 3.3, we find

$$a(\ell; \alpha(M, \ell)) < a(k; \alpha(k, k)) = a(k; \alpha) \tag{3.34}$$

for ℓ such that $2 \leq \ell < M \leq k$. By numerical calculation, we verify that (3.34) holds for $\alpha = 0.05, 0.01$, and $3 \leq k \leq 10$. From the construction of the closed testing procedure [3.3] and the relation of (3.34), we get the following (i) and (ii). (i) The procedure [3.3] of level α rejects $H_{(i,i')}$ that is rejected by the Tukey-Kramer type

Table 3.4 When $k = 4$, in testing the null hypothesis $H_{(1,2)}$ as a multiple comparison, the null hypotheses $H(I_1, \ldots, I_J) \in \mathscr{H}_{1(1,2)}$ that are tested as a closed testing procedure

M	$H(I_1, \ldots, I_J)$	J	ℓ
4	$H(\{1, 2, 3, 4\}) = H_0,$	$J = 1,$	$\ell_1 = 4$
	$H(\{1, 2\}, \{3, 4\}) :$	$J = 2,$	$\ell_1 = \ell_2 = 2$
	$p_1 = p_2, \ p_3 = p_4$		
3	$H(\{1, 2, 3\}) : p_1 =$	$J = 1,$	$\ell_1 = 3$
	$p_2 = p_3,$		
	$H(\{1, 2, 4\}) : p_1 =$	$J = 1,$	$\ell_1 = 3$
	$p_2 = p_4$		
2	$H(\{1, 2\}) : p_1 = p_2$	$J = 1,$	$\ell_1 = 2$

Table 3.5 When $k = 5$, in testing the null hypothesis $H_{(1,2)}$ as a multiple comparison, the null hypotheses $H(I_1, \ldots, I_J) \in \overline{\mathscr{H}}_{1(1,2)}$ that are tested as a closed testing procedure

M		$H(I_1, \ldots, I_J)$	
5	$H(\{1, 2, 3, 4, 5\}),$	$H(\{1, 2, 3\}, \{4, 5\}),$	$H(\{1, 2, 4\}, \{3, 5\}),$
	$H(\{1, 2, 5\}, \{3, 4\}),$	$H(\{1, 2\}, \{3, 4, 5\})$	
4	$H(\{1, 2, 3, 4\}),$	$H(\{1, 2, 3, 5\}),$	$H(\{1, 2, 4, 5\}),$
	$H(\{1, 2\}, \{3, 4\}),$	$H(\{1, 2\}, \{3, 5\}),$	$H(\{1, 2\}, \{4, 5\})$
3	$H(\{1, 2, 3\}),$	$H(\{1, 2, 4\}),$	$H(\{1, 2, 5\})$
2	$H(\{1, 2\})$		

$H(\{1, 2, 3, 4, 5\}) = H_0, \ J = 1, \ \ell_1 = 5$
$H(\{1, 2, 5\}, \{3, 4\}) : \ p_1 = p_2 = p_5, \ p_3 = p_4, \ J = 2, \ \ell_1 = 3, \ \ell_2 = 2$
$H(\{1, 2\}, \{3, 5\}) : \ p_1 = p_2, \ p_3 = p_5, \ J = 2, \ \ell_1 = 2, \ \ell_2 = 2$
$H(\{1, 2, 5\}) : \ p_1 = p_2 = p_5, \ J = 1, \ \ell_1 = 3$
$H(\{1, 2\}) = H_{(1,2)} : \ p_1 = p_2, \ J = 1, \ \ell_1 = 2$

simultaneous test [3.1] of level α. (ii) The Tukey-Kramer type simultaneous test [3.1] of level α does not always reject $H_{(i,i')}$ that is rejected by the procedure [3.3] of level α. Hence for $\alpha = 0.05, \ 0.01$, and $3 \leq k \leq 10$, the closed testing procedure [3.3] is more powerful than the single-step Tukey-Kramer type simultaneous test [3.1].

We get Lemma 3.1.

Lemma 3.1 *Let $A_{(i,i')}$ be the event that $H_{(i,i')}$ is rejected by the procedure [3.3] as a multiple comparison of level α ($(i, i') \in \mathcal{U}_k$). Suppose that*

$$a(\ell; \alpha(M, \ell)) < a(k; \alpha) \tag{3.35}$$

is satisfied for any M such that $4 \leq M \leq k$ and any integer ℓ such that $2 \leq \ell \leq M - 2$, where M is defined by (3.27). Then the following relations hold.

$$\bigcup_{(i,i')\in\mathcal{U}_k} A_{(i,i')} = \left\{\max_{(i,i')\in\mathcal{U}_k} |T_{i'i}| > a(k;\alpha)\right\}, \tag{3.36}$$

$$A_{(i,i')} \supset \{|T_{i'i}| > a(k;\alpha)\} \quad ((i,i')\in\mathcal{U}_k) \tag{3.37}$$

Proof For $(i,i')\in\mathcal{U}_k$, we put

$$B_{(i,i')} := \{|T_{i'i}| > a(k;\alpha)\}. \tag{3.38}$$

If $|T_{i'i}| > a(k;\alpha)$ is satisfied, by using (3.35), the procedure [3.3] of level α rejects $H_{(i,i')}$. This implies $B_{(i,i')} \subset A_{(i,i')}$. Hence we get (3.37) and

$$\bigcup_{(i,i')\in\mathcal{U}_k} B_{(i,i')} \subset \bigcup_{(i,i')\in\mathcal{U}_k} A_{(i,i')}. \tag{3.39}$$

If $H_{(i,i')}$ is rejected by the procedure [3.3] of level α, $\max_{(i,i')\in\mathcal{U}_k} |T_{i'i}| > a(k;\alpha)$ holds. Therefore we have

$$A_{(i,i')} \subset \bigcup_{(i,i')\in\mathcal{U}_k} B_{(i,i')}. \tag{3.40}$$

From (3.39) and (3.40), we get

$$\bigcup_{(i,i')\in\mathcal{U}_k} A_{(i,i')} = \bigcup_{(i,i')\in\mathcal{U}_k} B_{(i,i')}$$

which implies (3.36). $\qquad\square$

From a straightforward application of Lemma 3.1, we get Theorem 3.3.

Theorem 3.3 *Under the assumptions of Lemma 3.1, the following relations hold.*

$$P\left(\bigcup_{(i,i')\in\mathcal{U}_k} A_{(i,i')}\right) = P\left(\max_{(i,i')\in\mathcal{U}_k} |T_{i'i}| > a(k;\alpha)\right), \tag{3.41}$$

$$P\left(A_{(i,i')}\right) \geq P\left(|T_{i'i}| > a(k;\alpha)\right) \quad ((i,i')\in\mathcal{U}_k). \tag{3.42}$$

The left-hand side (L.H.S) of (3.41) is the probability that the procedure [3.3] rejects at least one of the hypotheses in $\mathcal{H}_1$. The right-hand side (R.H.S.) of (3.41) is the probability that the Tukey-Kramer type test rejects at least one of these hypotheses. The L.H.S. of (3.42) is the probability that the procedure [3.3] rejects $H_{(i,i')}$. The R.H.S. of (3.42) is the probability that the Tukey-Kramer type test rejects $H_{(i,i')}$. The relation (3.42) means that the L.H.S. is greater than or equal to the R.H.S. For any p, (3.41) and (3.42) hold.

As a closed testing procedure under assuming normality for k sample model, the REGW (Ryan–Einot–Gabriel–Welsch) method is utilized. The REGW method is also stated in Hsu (1996). In order to introduce the REGW type method in the k sample models with Bernoulli responses, we define the hypothesis $H(I)$ by $H(I)$: $p_i = p_{i'}$ for $i, i' \in I$ and we put $\iota := \#(I)$, where I ($I \subset \{1, \ldots, k\}$) and $\#(I) \geq 2$. Suppose $k \geq 4$. We define $\alpha^*(\iota)$ by

$$\alpha^*(\iota) = \begin{cases} 1 - (1-\alpha)^{\iota/k} & (2 \leq \iota \leq k-2) \\ \alpha & (\iota = k-1, k). \end{cases} \tag{3.43}$$

[3.4] REGW Type Method
If $a\,(\iota; \alpha^*(\iota)) < T(I)$ for any I such that $i, i' \in I$, $H_{(i,i')}$ is rejected.
   Suppose $\ell_j = \iota = \ell$. Then, since

$$1 - (1-\alpha)^{\ell/M} \geq 1 - (1-\alpha)^{\ell/k},$$

in testing the null hypothesis $\bigwedge_{v \in V} H_v$, the rejection region for the closed testing procedure [3.3] includes the one for the closed testing procedure [3.4]. Therefore, the closed testing procedure [3.3] is more powerful than the closed testing procedure [3.4].

   We propose stepwise procedure [3.5] based on the statistic S of (3.2).

[3.5] Stepwise Procedure Based on Asymptotic χ^2-Statistics
Let us put, for $j = 1, \ldots, J$,

$$S(I_j) := 4 \sum_{i \in I_j} n_i \left\{ \arcsin\left(\sqrt{\hat{p}_i}\right) - \sum_{i' \in I_j} \left(\frac{n_{i'}}{n(I_j)}\right) \arcsin\left(\sqrt{\hat{p}_{i'}}\right) \right\}^2, \tag{3.44}$$

where I_j is defined in (3.26) and $n(I_j) := \sum_{i \in I_j} n_i$. In the procedure [3.3], replace $a\left(\ell_j; \alpha(M, \ell_j)\right) < T(I_j)$ and $a\,(M; \alpha) < T(I_1)$ with $\chi^2_{\ell_j - 1}\left(\alpha(M, \ell_j)\right) < S(I_j)$ and $\chi^2_{M-1}(\alpha) < S(I_1)$, respectively. Here ℓ_j is defined in (3.27). Then, this procedure also becomes a closed test.

   For $\alpha = 0.05,\ 0.01$, we give the values of $\chi^2_\ell(\alpha(M, \ell))$ in Tables 3.6 and 3.7, respectively. We limited attention to $2 \leq M \leq 10$. $\ell = M - 1$ is not used in the procedure [3.5]. When $\ell = M = k$ is satisfied, $\chi^2_\ell(\alpha(M, \ell)) = \chi^2_k(\alpha)$ holds.

Table 3.6 The values of $\chi_{\ell-1}^2(\alpha(M, \ell))$ for the stepwise procedure [3.5] with $\alpha = 0.05$

$M \setminus \ell$	2	3	4	5	6	7	8	9	10
10	6.599	8.364	9.804	11.113	12.349	13.536	14.689	◊	16.919
9	6.412	8.155	9.576	10.868	12.087	13.259	◊	15.507	
8	6.205	7.921	9.320	10.592	11.793	◊	14.067		
7	5.970	7.657	9.031	10.279	◊	12.592			
6	5.701	7.352	8.696	◊	11.070				
5	5.385	6.993	◊	9.488					
4	5.002	◊	7.815						
3	◊	5.991							
2	3.841								

The places of ◊ are not used in the procedure [3.5]

Table 3.7 The values of $\chi_{\ell-1}^2(\alpha(M, \ell))$ for the stepwise procedure [3.5] with $\alpha = 0.01$

$M \setminus \ell$	2	3	4	5	6	7	8	9	10
10	9.542	11.611	13.310	14.855	16.310	17.706	19.058	◊	21.666
9	9.349	11.401	13.085	14.616	16.059	17.443	◊	20.090	
8	9.134	11.166	12.833	14.349	15.777	◊	18.475		
7	8.890	10.899	12.547	14.045	◊	16.812			
6	8.609	10.592	12.216	◊	15.086				
5	8.278	10.228	◊	13.277					
4	7.875	◊	11.345						
3	◊	9.210							
2	6.635								

References

Enderton HB (2001) A mathematical introduction to logic, 2nd edn. Academic, New York

Hayter AJ (1984) A proof of the conjecture that the Tukey-Kramer multiple comparisons procedure is conservative. Ann Stat 12:61–75

Hochberg Y, Tamhane AC (1987) Multiple comparison procedures. Wiley, New York

Hsu JC (1996) Multiple comparisons-theory and methods. Chapman & Hall, United Kingdom

Kramer CY (1956) Extension of multiple range tests to group means with unequal numbers of replications. Biometrics 12:307–310

Shiraishi T (2006) The upper bound for the distribution of Tukey-Kramer's statistic. Bull Comput Stat 19:77–87

Shiraishi T (2011a) Closed testing procedures for pairwise comparisons in multi-sample models. Biometric Soc Jpn 32:33–47 (in Japanese)

Shiraishi T (2011b) Multiple comparison procedures under continuous distributions. Kyoritsu-Shuppan Co. Ltd, Tokyo (in Japanese)

Shiraishi T, Matsuda S (2016) Closed testing procedures based on $\overline{\chi}^2$-statistics in multi-sample models with Bernoulli responses under simple ordered restrictions. Jpn J Biom 37:67–87

Shiraishi T, Sugiura H, Matsuda S (2019) Pairwise multiple comparisons-theory and computation. SpringerBriefs. Springer International Publishing, Berlin

Tukey JW (1953) The problem of multiple comparisons. The collected works of John W. Tukey (1994), Volume VIII: multiple comparisons. Chapman & Hall, United Kingdom

Chapter 4
Multiple Comparison Tests with a Control

Abstract The simultaneous confidence intervals for all pairwise differences among the proportions are expressed in Hochberg and Tamhane (1987) in k binomial populations. However, the degree of the conservativeness for the simultaneous confidence intervals depends on unknown proportion parameters. Therefore multiple tests based on arcsine transformation for all-pairwise comparison are proposed in Chap. 3. Chapter 3 shows that the degree of the conservativeness for the proposed tests is controlled by the sizes of the samples. For the multiple comparisons with a control, the multiple test procedures based on the Bonferroni inequality are stated in Shiraishi (2009), and Tanaka and Tarumi (1997). By using the arcsine transformation, it can be confirmed that the Dunnett-type multiple tests is superior to the former tests. Lastly a sequentially rejective procedure is discussed as a multi-step procedure.

4.1 Introduction

We consider k sample models with Bernoulli responses. $(X_{i1}, \ldots, X_{in_i})$ is a random sample of size n_i from the i-th Bernoulli population with success probability p_i $(i = 1, \ldots, k)$. It is convenient to assign the number 1 to a success and the number 0 to a failure. The settings for this model are same as in Sect. 2.1. Suppose that p_1 is the proportion of the control and $p_2, \ldots, p_k$ are the proportions of the new treatments.

For specified integer i such that $2 \leq i \leq k$, we want to test

$$\text{the null hypothesis } H_i : p_i = p_1. \tag{4.1}$$

For this null hypothesis, we may consider three alternative hypotheses as follows.

T. Shiraishi, *Multiple Comparisons for Bernoulli Data*,
JSS Research Series in Statistics,
https://doi.org/10.1007/978-981-19-2708-9_4

① Two-sided altenative hypothesis $H_i^{A\pm} : p_i \neq p_1$

② One-sided altenative hypothesis $H_i^{A+} : p_i > p_1$

③ One-sided altenative hypothesis $H_i^{A-} : p_i < p_1$.

In this chapter, we are interested in test procedures for three pairwise comparisons of $\{$the null hypothesis H_i versus the alternative $H_i^{A\pm} | i \in \mathscr{I}_{2,k}\}$, $\{$the null hypothesis H_i versus the alternative $H_i^{A+} | i \in \mathscr{I}_{2,k}\}$, and $\{$the null hypothesis H_i versus the alternative $H_i^{A-} | i \in \mathscr{I}_{2,k}\}$, where

$$\mathscr{I}_{2,k} := \{i \mid 2 \leq i \leq k\}. \tag{4.2}$$

Dunnett (1955) proposed single-step procedures as multiple comparison tests of level α in homoscedastic k sample model under normality.

Throughout this chapter, we suppose that the assumption of (A1) stated in Sect. 3.1 is satisfied.

Procedures and theory stated in this chapter are used in hybrid serial gatekeeping procedures for multiple comparisons with a control of Chap. 9.

4.2 The Single-Step Procedures

The estimator $\hat{p}_i$ for p_i is given by (3.5). We put, for $i = 2, \ldots, k$,

$$T_i(p) := \frac{2\left\{\arcsin\left(\sqrt{\hat{p}_i}\right) - \arcsin\left(\sqrt{\hat{p}_1}\right) - \arcsin\left(\sqrt{p_i}\right) + \arcsin\left(\sqrt{p_1}\right)\right\}}{\sqrt{\frac{1}{n_i} + \frac{1}{n_1}}}, \tag{4.3}$$

$$T_i := \frac{2\left\{\arcsin\left(\sqrt{\hat{p}_i}\right) - \arcsin\left(\sqrt{\hat{p}_1}\right)\right\}}{\sqrt{\frac{1}{n_i} + \frac{1}{n_1}}}, \tag{4.4}$$

$$\widetilde{T}_i(p) := \frac{\hat{p}_i - \hat{p}_1 - (p_i - p_1)}{\sqrt{\frac{1}{n_i}\hat{p}_i(1 - \hat{p}_i) + \frac{1}{n_1}\hat{p}_1(1 - \hat{p}_1)}}, \tag{4.5}$$

$$\widetilde{T}_i := \frac{\hat{p}_i - \hat{p}_1}{\sqrt{\frac{1}{n_i}\hat{p}_i(1 - \hat{p}_i) + \frac{1}{n_1}\hat{p}_1(1 - \hat{p}_1)}} \tag{4.6}$$

where $\boldsymbol{p} := (p_1, \ldots, p_k)$.

By using (3.10) and (3.11), we get Theorem 4.1.

Theorem 4.1 *For $t > 0$, under the assumption of (A1), we have*

$$\lim_{n\to\infty} P\left(\max_{2\leq i\leq k} |T_i(p)| \leq t\right) = \lim_{n\to\infty} P_0\left(\max_{2\leq i\leq k} |T_i| \leq t\right) = B_1(t|k,\boldsymbol{\lambda}), \quad (4.7)$$

$$\lim_{n\to\infty} P\left(\max_{2\leq i\leq k} T_i(p) \leq t\right) = \lim_{n\to\infty} P_0\left(\max_{2\leq i\leq k} T_i \leq t\right) = B_2(t|k,\boldsymbol{\lambda}), \quad (4.8)$$

$$\lim_{n\to\infty} P\left(\max_{2\leq i\leq k} |\widetilde{T}_i(p)| \leq t\right) = \widetilde{B}_1(t|k,\boldsymbol{q}), \quad (4.9)$$

$$\lim_{n\to\infty} P\left(\max_{2\leq i\leq k} |\widetilde{T}_i(p)| \leq t\right) \neq \lim_{n\to\infty} P_0\left(\max_{2\leq i\leq k} |\widetilde{T}_i| \leq t\right), \quad (4.10)$$

$$\lim_{n\to\infty} P\left(\max_{2\leq i\leq k} \widetilde{T}_i(p) \leq t\right) = \widetilde{B}_2(t|k,\boldsymbol{q}), \quad (4.11)$$

$$\lim_{n\to\infty} P\left(\max_{2\leq i\leq k} \widetilde{T}_i(p) \leq t\right) \neq \lim_{n\to\infty} P_0\left(\max_{2\leq i\leq k} \widetilde{T}_i \leq t\right), \quad (4.12)$$

where $P_0(\cdot)$ stands for the probability measure under the null hypothesis H_0 of (3.1),

$$B_1(t|k,\boldsymbol{\lambda}) := \int_{-\infty}^{\infty} \prod_{i=2}^{k} \left\{ \Phi\left(\sqrt{\frac{\lambda_i}{\lambda_1}}\cdot x + \sqrt{\frac{\lambda_i + \lambda_1}{\lambda_1}}\cdot t\right) \right.$$
$$\left. - \Phi\left(\sqrt{\frac{\lambda_i}{\lambda_1}}\cdot x - \sqrt{\frac{\lambda_i + \lambda_1}{\lambda_1}}\cdot t\right) \right\} d\Phi(x),$$

$$B_2(t|k,\boldsymbol{\lambda}) := \int_{-\infty}^{\infty} \prod_{i=2}^{k} \Phi\left(\sqrt{\frac{\lambda_i}{\lambda_1}}\cdot x + \sqrt{\frac{\lambda_i + \lambda_1}{\lambda_1}}\cdot t\right) d\Phi(x),$$

$$\widetilde{B}_1(t|k,\boldsymbol{q}) := \int_{-\infty}^{\infty} \prod_{i=2}^{k} \left\{ \Phi\left(\sqrt{\frac{q_1}{q_i}}\cdot x + \sqrt{\frac{q_i + q_1}{q_i}}\cdot t\right) \right.$$
$$\left. - \Phi\left(\sqrt{\frac{q_1}{q_i}}\cdot x - \sqrt{\frac{q_i + q_1}{q_i}}\cdot t\right) \right\} d\Phi(x),$$

$$\widetilde{B}_2(t|k,\boldsymbol{q}) := \int_{-\infty}^{\infty} \prod_{i=2}^{k} \Phi\left(\sqrt{\frac{q_1}{q_i}}\cdot x + \sqrt{\frac{q_i + q_1}{q_i}}\cdot t\right) d\Phi(x),$$

$\boldsymbol{\lambda}$ and $\boldsymbol{q}$ are defined by (3.18), and q_i is defined by (3.19). □

For a given α such that $0 < \alpha < 1$, we put

Table 4.1 The values of $b_1(k, 1/k, \ldots, 1/k; \alpha)$ for $n_1 = \ldots = n_k$

$100\alpha\%$ \ k	2	3	4	5	6	7	8	9	10
5%	1.960	2.212	2.349	2.442	2.511	2.567	2.613	2.652	2.686
1%	2.576	2.794	2.915	2.998	3.060	3.110	3.152	3.188	3.219

Table 4.2 The values of $b_2(k, 1/k, \ldots, 1/k; \alpha)$ for $n_1 = \ldots = n_k$

$100\alpha\%$ \ k	2	3	4	5	6	7	8	9	10
5%	1.645	1.916	2.062	2.160	2.234	2.292	2.340	2.381	2.417
1%	2.326	2.558	2.685	2.772	2.837	2.889	2.933	2.970	3.002

$$b_1(k, \lambda_1, \ldots, \lambda_k; \alpha)$$
$$:= \text{a solution of } t \text{ satisfying the equation } B_1(t|k, \boldsymbol{\lambda}) = 1 - \alpha, \qquad (4.13)$$
$$b_2(k, \lambda_1, \ldots, \lambda_k; \alpha)$$
$$:= \text{a solution of } t \text{ satisfying the equation } B_2(t|k, \boldsymbol{\lambda}) = 1 - \alpha. \qquad (4.14)$$

For $\alpha = 0.05$, 0.01, we give the values of $b_1(k, 1/k, \ldots, 1/k; \alpha)$ and $b_2(k, 1/k, \ldots, 1/k; \alpha)$ in Tables 4.1 and 4.2, respectively. We limited attention to $2 \le k \le 10$.

From (4.7) and (4.8) of Theorem 4.1, we get asymptotic simultaneous tests of [4.1].

[4.1] Dunnett Type Tests Based on Arcsine Transformation

(1) The Dunnett type test of level α for {the null hypothesis H_i versus the alternative $H_i^{A\pm} \big| i \in \mathscr{I}_{2,k}$} consists in rejecting H_i for $i \in \mathscr{I}_{2,k}$ such that $|T_i| > b_1(k, \lambda_1, \ldots, \lambda_k; \alpha)$.

(2) The Dunnett type test of level α for {the null hypothesis H_i versus the alternative $H_i^{A+} \big| i \in \mathscr{I}_{2,k}$} consists in rejecting H_i for $i \in \mathscr{I}_{2,k}$ such that $T_i > b_2(k, \lambda_1, \ldots, \lambda_k; \alpha)$.

(3) The Dunnett type test of level α for {the null hypothesis H_i versus the alternative $H_i^{A-} \big| i \in \mathscr{I}_{2,k}$} consists in rejecting H_i for $i \in \mathscr{I}_{2,k}$ such that $-T_i > b_2(k, \lambda_1, \ldots, \lambda_k; \alpha)$.

4.3   Closed Testing Procedures

Let us put
$$\mathscr{H}_2 := \{H_2, \ldots, H_k\} = \{H_i \,|\, i \in \mathscr{I}_{2,k}\}. \qquad (4.15)$$

Then, the closure of $\mathscr{H}_2$ is given by

$$\overline{\mathscr{H}}_2 := \left\{ \bigwedge_{i \in E} H_i \ \middle| \ \emptyset \subsetneqq E \subset \mathscr{I}_{2,k} \right\}.$$

For E such that $E \subset \mathscr{I}_{2,k}$, let us define the hypothesis that $p_i = p_1$ for $i \in E$ by $H(E)$. Then

$$\bigwedge_{i \in E} H_i = H(E)$$

holds.

[4.2] Multi-step Procedure

Take the specific null hypothesis $H_{i_0} \in \mathscr{H}_2$. Then the closed testing procedure is to reject H_{i_0} if the test of the null hypothesis $H(E)$ is rejected at level α for any E that satisfies $i_0 \in E \subset \mathscr{I}_{2,k}$.

We put $\ell := \ell(E) := \#(E)$,

$$E := \{i_1, \dots, i_\ell\} \quad (2 \le i_1 < \cdots < i_\ell \le k), \tag{4.16}$$

$$B_1(t|\ell + 1, E) := \int_{-\infty}^{\infty} \prod_{j=1}^{\ell} \left\{ \Phi\left(\sqrt{\frac{\lambda_{i_j}}{\lambda_1}} \cdot x + \sqrt{\frac{\lambda_{i_j} + \lambda_1}{\lambda_1}} \cdot t \right) \right.$$
$$\left. - \Phi\left(\sqrt{\frac{\lambda_{i_j}}{\lambda_1}} \cdot x - \sqrt{\frac{\lambda_{i_j} + \lambda_1}{\lambda_1}} \cdot t \right) \right\} d\Phi(x), \tag{4.17}$$

and

$$B_2(t|\ell + 1, E) := \int_{-\infty}^{\infty} \prod_{j=1}^{\ell} \Phi\left(\sqrt{\frac{\lambda_{i_j}}{\lambda_1}} \cdot x + \sqrt{\frac{\lambda_{i_j} + \lambda_1}{\lambda_1}} \cdot t \right) d\Phi(x). \tag{4.18}$$

Further, for a given α such that $0 < \alpha < 1$, we put

$b_1(\ell + 1, \lambda_1, \lambda_{i_1}, \dots, \lambda_{i_\ell}; \alpha)$
    $:= $ a solution of t satisfying the equation $B_1(t|\ell + 1, E) = 1 - \alpha$, (4.19)
$b_2(\ell + 1, \lambda_1, \lambda_{i_1}, \dots, \lambda_{i_\ell}; \alpha)$
    $:= $ a solution of t satisfying the equation $B_2(t|\ell + 1, E) = 1 - \alpha$. (4.20)

Then we have

$$\lim_{n \to \infty} P_0 \left(\max_{i \in E} |T_i| > b_1(\ell + 1, \lambda_1, \lambda_{i_1}, \dots, \lambda_{i_\ell}; \alpha) \right) = \alpha,$$

$$\lim_{n \to \infty} P_0 \left(\max_{i \in E} T_i > b_2(\ell + 1, , \lambda_1, \lambda_{i_1}, \dots, \lambda_{i_\ell}; \alpha) \right) = \alpha.$$

(1) The multiple comparison test for {the null hypothesis H_i versus the alternative $H_i^{A\pm} \big| i \in \mathscr{I}_{2,k}$}:
    If $\max_{i \in E} |T_i| > b_1(\ell + 1, , \lambda_1, \lambda_{i_1}, \dots, \lambda_{i_\ell}; \alpha)$, $H(E)$ is rejected.

(2) The multiple comparison test for {the null hypothesis H_i versus the alternative $H_i^{A+} \big| i \in \mathscr{I}_{2,k}$}:
    If $\max_{i \in E} T_i > b_2(\ell + 1, , \lambda_1, \lambda_{i_1}, \dots, \lambda_{i_\ell}; \alpha)$, $H(E)$ is rejected.

(3) The multiple comparison test for {the null hypothesis H_i versus the alternative $H_i^{A-} \big| i \in \mathscr{I}_{2,k}$}:
    If $\max_{i \in E}(-T_i) > b_2(\ell + 1, , \lambda_1, \lambda_{i_1}, \dots, \lambda_{i_\ell}; \alpha)$, $H(E)$ is rejected.

Next we introduce sequentially rejective multiple test procedures. For simplicity, we assume $\lambda_2 = \dots = \lambda_k$. $B_1(t|\ell + 1, E)$ of (4.17) and $B_2(t|\ell + 1, E)$ of (4.18) become

$$B_1(t|\ell + 1, E) = \int_{-\infty}^{\infty} \left\{ \Phi\left(\sqrt{\frac{\lambda_2}{\lambda_1}} \cdot x + \sqrt{1 + \frac{\lambda_2}{\lambda_1}} \cdot t \right) \right.$$
$$\left. - \Phi\left(\sqrt{\frac{\lambda_2}{\lambda_1}} \cdot x - \sqrt{1 + \frac{\lambda_2}{\lambda_1}} \cdot t \right) \right\}^{\ell} d\Phi(x) \quad (4.21)$$

and

$$B_2(t|\ell + 1, E) = \int_{-\infty}^{\infty} \left\{ \Phi\left(\sqrt{\frac{\lambda_2}{\lambda_1}} \cdot x + \sqrt{1 + \frac{\lambda_2}{\lambda_1}} \cdot t \right) \right\}^{\ell} d\Phi(x). \quad (4.22)$$

We put

$$b^*(\ell + 1, \lambda_1, \lambda_2; \alpha) := \begin{cases} b_1(\ell + 1, , \lambda_1, \lambda_2, \dots, \lambda_2; \alpha) & (H_i^{A\pm} \text{ is alternative}) \\ b_2(\ell + 1, , \lambda_1, \lambda_2, \dots, \lambda_2; \alpha) & (H_i^{A+} \text{ is alternative}) \\ b_2(\ell + 1, , \lambda_1, \lambda_2, \dots, \lambda_2; \alpha) & (H_i^{A-} \text{ is alternative}) \end{cases}$$

and

$$T_i^* := \begin{cases} |T_i| & (H_i^{A\pm} \text{ is alternative}) \\ T_i & (H_i^{A+} \text{ is alternative}) \\ -T_i & (H_i^{A-} \text{ is alternative}). \end{cases}$$

Let $T_{(1)}^* \leq T_{(2)}^* \leq \dots \leq T_{(k-1)}^*$ be the ordered statistics of T_i^*'s and let $H_{(1)}, \dots, H_{(k-1)}$ be the corresponding hypotheses. Then we get multi-step procedures [4.3].

[4.3] Sequentially Rejective Multiple Test Procedures

For ℓ such that $1 \leq \ell \leq k - 1$, we proceed as follows.

(Step 1) We put $\ell = k - 1$.

(Step 2)

   (i) If $T_{(\ell)}^* \leq b^*(\ell + 1, \lambda_1, \lambda_2; \alpha)$, $H_{(1)}, \ldots, H_{(\ell)}$ are not rejected. Finish this test procedure.

   (ii) If $T_{(\ell)}^* > b^*(\ell + 1, \lambda_1, \lambda_2; \alpha)$, H_ℓ is rejected and go to step 3.

(Step 3)

   (i) When $\ell \geq 2$, set $\ell - 1$ as ℓ and return step 2.

   (ii) When $\ell = 1$, finish this test procedure.   □

The multi-step procedures of [4.2] and [4.3] are more powerful than the single-step procedure [4.1].

References

Dunnett CW (1955) A multiple comparison procedure for comparing several treatments with a control. J Am Stat Assoc 50:1096–1121

Hochberg Y, Tamhane AC (1987) Multiple comparison procedures. Wiley, New York

Shiraishi T (2009) Simultaneous confidence intervals based on logarithm transformations in multi-sample models with Bernoulli responses. Japanes J Appl Stat 38:135–150 (in Japanese)

Tanaka Y, Tarumi T (1997) Handbook of statistical analysis. Kyoritsu-Shuppan Co. Ltd, Tokyo (in Japanese)

Chapter 5
Simultaneous Confidence Intervals

Abstract In Chap. 3, we state multiple tests for all-pairwise comparison tests. In Chap. 4, we state multiple comparison tests with a control. In the present chapter, we discuss simultaneous confidence intervals for all the pairwise differences among the proportions and differences with a control. Furthermore, we discuss simultaneous confidence intervals for all-pairwise odds ratios and relative risks.

5.1 Introduction

We consider k-sample models with Bernoulli responses. $(X_{i1}, \ldots, X_{in_i})$ is a random sample of size n_i from the i-th Bernoulli population with success probability p_i $(i = 1, \ldots, k)$. It is convenient to assign the number 1 to a success and the number 0 to a failure. The settings for this model are same as in Sect. 2.1.

Throughout this chapter, we suppose that the assumption of (A1) stated in Sect. 3.1 is satisfied.

5.2 Pairwise Differences of Proportions Based on Arcsine Transformation

Suppose that $g(\cdot)$ is a given real-valued function and $I_{(i',i)}$ is an interval for any $(i, i') \in \mathscr{U}_k$, where $\mathscr{U}_k$ is defined by (3.4). If

$$\lim_{n \to \infty} P\left(\text{For any } (i, i') \in \mathscr{U}_k, \ g(p_{i'}) - g(p_i) \in I_{(i',i)}\right) \geq 1 - \alpha,$$

we refer to $g(p_{i'}) - g(p_i) \in I_{(i',i)}$ $((i, i') \in \mathscr{U}_k)$ as asymptotic $100(1 - \alpha)\%$ simultaneous confidence intervals for $\{g(p_{i'}) - g(p_i) \mid (i, i') \in \mathscr{U}_k\}$. From the left-hand

T. Shiraishi, *Multiple Comparisons for Bernoulli Data*,
JSS Research Series in Statistics,
https://doi.org/10.1007/978-981-19-2708-9_5

side of the inequalities in (3.12) of Theorem 3.1, we get the asymptotic simultaneous confidence intervals of [5.1].

[5.1] Tukey-Kramer-Type Simultaneous Intervals Based on Arcsine Transformation

The asymptotic $100(1 - \alpha)\%$ simultaneous confidence intervals for $\{\arcsin\left(\sqrt{p_{i'}}\right) - \arcsin\left(\sqrt{p_i}\right) \mid (i, i') \in \mathscr{U}_k\}$ are given by

$$\arcsin\left(\sqrt{\hat{p}_{i'}}\right) - \arcsin\left(\sqrt{\hat{p}_i}\right) - a(k; \alpha) \cdot \sqrt{\frac{1}{4n_i} + \frac{1}{4n_{i'}}}$$

$$< \arcsin\left(\sqrt{p_{i'}}\right) - \arcsin\left(\sqrt{p_i}\right)$$

$$< \arcsin\left(\sqrt{\hat{p}_{i'}}\right) - \arcsin\left(\sqrt{\hat{p}_i}\right) + a(k; \alpha) \cdot \sqrt{\frac{1}{4n_i} + \frac{1}{4n_{i'}}} \quad ((i, i') \in \mathscr{U}_k).$$

Here, $a(k; \alpha)$ is defined by (3.20) and the values of $a(k; \alpha)$ for $\alpha = 0.05, 0.01$ and $2 \leq k \leq 10$ are given by Table 3.1. Although the simultaneous confidence intervals of [5.1] are conservative methods, the conservativeness is small.

From (4.7) and (4.8) of theorem 4.1, we get the asymptotic simultaneous confidence intervals of [5.2].

[5.2] Dunnett-Type Simultaneous Intervals Based on Arcsine Transformation

(1) The asymptotic $100(1 - \alpha)\%$ two-sided simultaneous confidence intervals for $\{\arcsin\left(\sqrt{p_i}\right) - \arcsin\left(\sqrt{p_1}\right) \mid i \in \mathscr{I}_{2,k}\}$ are given by

$$\arcsin\left(\sqrt{\hat{p}_i}\right) - \arcsin\left(\sqrt{\hat{p}_1}\right) - b_1(k, \lambda_1, \ldots, \lambda_k; \alpha) \cdot \sqrt{\frac{1}{4n_i} + \frac{1}{4n_1}}$$

$$< \arcsin\left(\sqrt{p_i}\right) - \arcsin\left(\sqrt{p_1}\right)$$

$$< \arcsin\left(\sqrt{\hat{p}_i}\right) - \arcsin\left(\sqrt{\hat{p}_1}\right) + b_1(k, \lambda_1, \ldots, \lambda_k; \alpha) \cdot \sqrt{\frac{1}{4n_i} + \frac{1}{4n_1}}$$

$$(i \in \mathscr{I}_{2,k}),$$

where $\mathscr{I}_{2,k}$ is defined by (4.2).

(2) The asymptotic $100(1 - \alpha)\%$ simultaneous lower confidence intervals for $\{\arcsin\left(\sqrt{p_i}\right) - \arcsin\left(\sqrt{p_1}\right) \mid i \in \mathscr{I}_{2,k}\}$ are given by

$$\arcsin\left(\sqrt{\hat{p}_i}\right) - \arcsin\left(\sqrt{\hat{p}_1}\right) - b_2(k, \lambda_1, \ldots, \lambda_k; \alpha) \cdot \sqrt{\frac{1}{4n_i} + \frac{1}{4n_1}}$$

$$< \arcsin\left(\sqrt{p_i}\right) - \arcsin\left(\sqrt{p_1}\right) < \frac{\pi}{2} \quad (i \in \mathscr{I}_{2,k}).$$

(3) The asymptotic $100(1 - \alpha)\%$ simultaneous upper confidence intervals for $\{\arcsin\left(\sqrt{p_i}\right) - \arcsin\left(\sqrt{p_1}\right) \mid i \in \mathcal{I}_{2,k}\}$ are given by

$$-\frac{\pi}{2} < \arcsin\left(\sqrt{p_i}\right) - \arcsin\left(\sqrt{p_1}\right)$$

$$< \arcsin\left(\sqrt{\hat{p}_i}\right) - \arcsin\left(\sqrt{\hat{p}_1}\right) + b_2(k, \lambda_1, \ldots, \lambda_k; \alpha) \cdot \sqrt{\frac{1}{4n_i} + \frac{1}{4n_1}}$$

$$(i \in \mathcal{I}_{2,k}).$$

Here, $b_1(k, \lambda_1, \ldots, \lambda_k; \alpha)$ and $b_2(k, \lambda_1, \ldots, \lambda_k; \alpha)$ are defined by (4.13) and (4.14). Their values are given by Tables 4.1 and 4.2.

It is not possible to construct Dunnett-type simultaneous intervals for $\{p_i - p_1 \mid i \in \mathcal{I}_{2,k}\}$.

5.3 All-Pairwise Differences of Proportions

From the left-hand side of the inequalities in (3.14) of Theorem 3.1, we may get the asymptotic simultaneous confidence intervals of [5.3].

[5.3] Tukey-Kramer-Type Simultaneous Intervals

The asymptotic $100(1 - \alpha)\%$ simultaneous confidence intervals for $\{p_{i'} - p_i \mid (i, i') \in \mathcal{U}_k\}$ are given by

$$\hat{p}_{i'} - \hat{p}_i - a(k; \alpha) \cdot \widetilde{SD}_{ii'} < p_{i'} - p_i < \hat{p}_{i'} - \hat{p}_i + a(k; \alpha) \cdot \widetilde{SD}_{ii'} \quad ((i, i') \in \mathcal{U}_k), \tag{5.1}$$

where $\widetilde{SD}_{ii'} := \sqrt{\frac{1}{n_i}\hat{p}_i(1 - \hat{p}_i) + \frac{1}{n_{i'}}\hat{p}_{i'}(1 - \hat{p}_{i'})}$.

[5.3] is stated in Hochberg and Tamhane (1987). Since the right-hand side of the inequalities in (3.14) of Theorem 3.1 depends on the unknown parameter p_i's, the upper bound for conservativeness of [5.3] is not solved. Although $-1 < p_{i'} - p_i < 1$ holds, the intervals of (5.1) may include -1 or 1. Thus, we consider logit transformation

$$\theta_{i'i} := \log\left\{\frac{\frac{p_{i'} - p_i + 1}{2}}{1 - \frac{p_{i'} - p_i + 1}{2}}\right\} = \log\left\{\frac{p_{i'} - p_i + 1}{1 - (p_{i'} - p_i)}\right\}$$

which implies

$$p_{i'} - p_i = \frac{e^{\theta_{i'i}} - 1}{e^{\theta_{i'i}} + 1}. \tag{5.2}$$

We may derive

$$c_{i'i} := \frac{d\theta_{i'i}}{d(p_{i'} - p_i)} = \frac{1}{1 + p_{i'} - p_i} + \frac{1}{1 - (p_{i'} - p_i)} = \frac{2}{1 - (p_{i'} - p_i)^2}. \quad (5.3)$$

Furthermore, we put

$$\hat{\theta}_{i'i} := \log \left\{ \frac{\hat{p}_{i'} - \hat{p}_i + 1}{1 - (\hat{p}_{i'} - \hat{p}_i)} \right\}.$$

From (3.10), we have

$$\sqrt{n}(\hat{p}_i - p_i) \xrightarrow{\mathscr{L}} Y_i \sim N \left(0, \frac{p_i(1 - p_i)}{\lambda_i} \right).$$

Since $Y_1, \ldots, Y_k$ is independent, we get

$$\sqrt{n}(\hat{p}_{i'} - \hat{p}_i - p_{i'} + p_i) \xrightarrow{\mathscr{L}} Y_{i'} - Y_i.$$

By the delta method, we may derive

$$\sqrt{n}(\hat{\theta}_{i'i} - \theta_{i'i}) \xrightarrow{\mathscr{L}} c_{i'i}(Y_{i'} - Y_i) \sim N \left(0, \frac{c_{ii'}^2 p_i(1 - p_i)}{\lambda_i} + \frac{c_{ii'}^2 p_{i'}(1 - p_{i'})}{\lambda_{i'}} \right).$$

$$(5.4)$$

For $\boldsymbol{p} := (p_1, \ldots, p_k)$, let us put

$$\widehat{T}_{i'i}(\boldsymbol{p}) := \frac{\{1 - (\hat{p}_{i'} - \hat{p}_i)^2\}(\hat{\theta}_{i'i} - \theta_{i'i})}{2\sqrt{\frac{1}{n_i}\hat{p}_i(1 - \hat{p}_i) + \frac{1}{n_{i'}}\hat{p}_{i'}(1 - \hat{p}_{i'})}}.$$

Then, from (5.4), we get

$$\widehat{T}_{i'i}(\boldsymbol{p}) \xrightarrow{\mathscr{L}} \frac{Y_{i'} - Y_i}{\sqrt{q_i + q_{i'}}}, \quad (5.5)$$

where q_i's are defined by (3.19). Hence, we find

$$\lim_{n \to \infty} P \left(\max_{1 \le i < i' \le k} |\widehat{T}_{i'i}(\boldsymbol{p})| \le t \right) = P \left(\max_{1 \le i < i' \le k} \left| \frac{Y_{i'} - Y_i}{\sqrt{q_i + q_{i'}}} \right| \le t \right).$$

We get the following result similar to (3.14) of Theorem 3.1.

$$A(t|k) \le \lim_{n \to \infty} P \left(\max_{1 \le i < i' \le k} |\widehat{T}_{i'i}(\boldsymbol{p})| \le t \right) \le A^*(t|k, \boldsymbol{q}), \quad (5.6)$$

where $A^*(t|k, \boldsymbol{q})$ and q_i are defined by (3.17) and (3.19). Hence, from the left-hand side of the inequalities in (5.6), the asymptotic $100(1 - \alpha)\%$ simultaneous confidence intervals for $\theta_{i'i}$ $((i, i') \in \mathscr{U}_k)$ are given by

$$\hat{\theta}_{i'i} - a(k;\alpha) \cdot \widehat{SD}_{ii'} < \theta_{i'i} < \hat{\theta}_{i'i} + a(k;\alpha) \cdot \widehat{SD}_{ii'} \quad ((i,i') \in \mathcal{U}_k), \qquad (5.7)$$

where

$$\widehat{SD}_{ii'} := \frac{2}{\{1 - (\hat{p}_{i'} - \hat{p}_i)^2\}} \cdot \sqrt{\frac{1}{n_i}\hat{p}_i(1-\hat{p}_i) + \frac{1}{n_{i'}}\hat{p}_{i'}(1-\hat{p}_{i'})} \quad ((i,i') \in \mathcal{U}_k).$$

We may get the asymptotic simultaneous confidence intervals of [5.4] which is equivalent to (5.7).

[5.4] Simultaneous Intervals Based on Logit Transformation
The asymptotic $100(1-\alpha)\%$ simultaneous confidence intervals for $\{p_{i'} - p_i \mid (i,i') \in \mathcal{U}_k\}$ are given by

$$\frac{\exp\{\hat{\theta}_{i'i} - a(k;\alpha) \cdot \widehat{SD}_{ii'}\} - 1}{\exp\{\hat{\theta}_{i'i} - a(k;\alpha) \cdot \widehat{SD}_{ii'}\} + 1} < p_{i'} - p_i < \frac{\exp\{\hat{\theta}_{i'i} + a(k;\alpha) \cdot \widehat{SD}_{ii'}\} - 1}{\exp\{\hat{\theta}_{i'i} + a(k;\alpha) \cdot \widehat{SD}_{ii'}\} + 1}$$
$$(5.8)$$
$$((i,i') \in \mathcal{U}_k).$$

Equation (5.8) do not include -1 and 1. Since conservativeness for [5.3] and [5.4] depends on unknown parameters q_i's, the degree of the conservativeness cannot be controlled.

5.4 Odds Ratios and Relative Risks of Proportions

Let us put

$$\theta_i := \log\left(\frac{p_i}{1 - p_i}\right).$$

Then we get

$$\frac{p_{i'}/(1 - p_{i'})}{p_i/(1 - p_i)} = \exp(\theta_{i'} - \theta_i) \text{ and } c_i := \frac{d\theta_i}{dp_i} = \frac{1}{p_i} + \frac{1}{1 - p_i} = \frac{1}{p_i(1 - p_i)}.$$

Furthermore, we put

$$\hat{\theta}_i := \log\left(\frac{\hat{p}_i}{1 - \hat{p}_i}\right). \qquad (5.9)$$

From the delta method, we have

$$\sqrt{n}(\hat{\theta}_i - \theta_i) \xrightarrow{\mathscr{L}} c_i Y_i \sim N\left(0, \frac{1}{\lambda_i p_i(1 - p_i)}\right). \qquad (5.10)$$

Thus, we get

$$\sqrt{n}\{(\hat{\theta}_{i'} - \hat{\theta}_i) - (\theta_{i'} - \theta_i)\} \xrightarrow{\mathcal{L}} c_{i'} Y_{i'} - c_i Y_i$$

$$\sim N\left(0, \frac{1}{\lambda_i p_i (1 - p_i)} + \frac{1}{\lambda_{i'} p_{i'} (1 - p_{i'})}\right). \quad (5.11)$$

For $p := (p_1, \ldots, p_k)$ and $(i, i') \in \mathcal{U}_k$, we put

$$\widehat{T}_{i'i}^{or}(p) := \frac{(\hat{\theta}_{i'} - \hat{\theta}_i) - (\theta_{i'} - \theta_i)}{\sqrt{\frac{1}{n_i \hat{p}_i (1 - \hat{p}_i)} + \frac{1}{n_{i'} \hat{p}_{i'} (1 - \hat{p}_{i'})}}}.$$

For $t > 0$, we get the following result similar to (5.6).

$$A(t|k) \leq \lim_{n \to \infty} P\left(\max_{1 \leq i < i' \leq k} |\widehat{T}_{i'i}^{or}(p)| \leq t\right) \leq A^*(t|k, q), \quad (5.12)$$

where $A^*(t|k, q)$ is defined by (3.17) and $q_i := 1/\{\lambda_i p_i (1 - p_i)\}$ $(i = 1, \ldots, k)$. Hence, from the left-hand side of the inequalities in (5.12), the asymptotic $100(1 - \alpha)\%$ simultaneous confidence intervals for $\theta_{i'} - \theta i$ $((i, i') \in \mathcal{U}_k)$ are given by

$$\hat{\theta}_{i'} - \hat{\theta}_i - a(k; \alpha) \cdot \widehat{SD}_{ii'}^{or} < \theta_{i'} - \theta_i < \hat{\theta}_{i'} - \hat{\theta}_i + a(k; \alpha) \cdot \widehat{SD}_{ii'}^{or} \quad ((i, i') \in \mathcal{U}_k),$$
$$(5.13)$$

where

$$\widehat{SD}_{ii'}^{or} := \sqrt{\frac{1}{n_i \hat{p}_i (1 - \hat{p}_i)} + \frac{1}{n_{i'} \hat{p}_{i'} (1 - \hat{p}_{i'})}}.$$

We may get the asymptotic simultaneous confidence intervals of [5.5] which is equivalent to (5.13).

[5.5] Simultaneous Intervals for Odds Ratios
The asymptotic $100(1 - \alpha)\%$ simultaneous confidence intervals for $\left\{\frac{p_{i'}/(1 - p_{i'})}{p_i/(1 - p_i)} \mid (i, i') \in \mathcal{U}_k\right\}$ are given by

$$\exp\left\{\hat{\theta}_{i'} - \hat{\theta}_i - a(k; \alpha) \cdot \widehat{SD}_{ii'}^{or}\right\} < \frac{p_{i'}/(1 - p_{i'})}{p_i/(1 - p_i)} < \exp\left\{\hat{\theta}_{i'} - \hat{\theta}_i + a(k; \alpha) \cdot \widehat{SD}_{ii'}^{or}\right\}$$

$$((i, i') \in \mathcal{U}_k).$$

Let us put

$$\widehat{T}_{i'i}^{rr}(p) := \frac{(\hat{\theta}_{i'}^* - \hat{\theta}_i^*) - (\theta_{i'}^* - \theta_i^*)}{\sqrt{\frac{1 - \hat{p}_i}{n_i \hat{p}_i} + \frac{1 - \hat{p}_{i'}}{n_{i'} \hat{p}_{i'}}}},$$

where $\theta_i^* := \log(p_i)$ and $\hat{\theta}_i^* := \log(\hat{p}_i)$ For $t > 0$, we get the following result similar to (5.12).

$$A(t|k) \leq \lim_{n \to \infty} P \left(\max_{1 \leq i < i' \leq k} |\widehat{T}_{i'i}^{rr}(\boldsymbol{p})| \leq t \right) \leq A^*(t|k, \boldsymbol{q}),$$

where $A^*(t|k, \boldsymbol{q})$ is defined by (3.17) and $q_i := (1 - p_i)/(\lambda_i p_i)$ $(i = 1, \ldots, k)$.

Hence, we may get the asymptotic simultaneous confidence intervals of [5.6] similar to [5.5].

[5.6] Simultaneous Intervals for Relative Risks

The asymptotic $100(1 - \alpha)\%$ simultaneous confidence intervals for $\{p_{i'}/p_i \mid (i, i') \in \mathcal{U}_k\}$ are given by

$$\exp\left\{\hat{\theta}_{i'}^* - \hat{\theta}_i^* - a(k; \alpha) \cdot \widehat{SD}_{ii'}^{rr}\right\} < \frac{p_{i'}}{p_i} < \exp\left\{\hat{\theta}_{i'}^* - \hat{\theta}_i^* + a(k; \alpha) \cdot \widehat{SD}_{ii'}^{rr}\right\} \quad ((i, i') \in \mathcal{U}_k),$$

where

$$\widehat{SD}_{ii'}^{rr} := \sqrt{\frac{1 - \hat{p}_i}{n_i \hat{p}_i} + \frac{1 - \hat{p}_{i'}}{n_{i'} \hat{p}_{i'}}}.$$

Reference

Hochberg Y, Tamhane AC (1987) Multiple comparison procedures. Wiley, New York

Chapter 6
All-Pairwise Comparisons Under Simple Order Restrictions

Abstract Multiple comparison procedures provide differences among the groups that are of interest. We consider a multi-sample model with Bernoulli responses under simple order restrictions of proportions. For all-pairwise comparisons, we discuss (i) closed testing procedures based on maximum values of two-sample test statistics and (ii) closed testing procedures based on statistics having asymptotically a $\bar{\chi}^2$−distribution which appeared in Chernoff (1954). The closed testing procedures of (ii) are applicable for the models with unequal sample sizes. Although single-step multiple comparison procedures are utilized in general, the power of these procedures is low for a large number of groups. The closed testing procedures are more powerful than the single-step procedures.

6.1 Introduction

In many applications of k-sample models for comparing proportions in clinical trials or experimental studies, individuals are classified as two possible outcomes, "success" and "failure". Let $p_1, \ldots, p_k$ correspond to the probabilities that individuals at each of k levels of treatment possess "success". For this setting, Agresti and Coull (1996) assumed k-sample Bernoulli responses models with the simple order restrictions

$$p_1 \le p_2 \le \ldots \le p_k. \tag{6.1}$$

For the k-sample models, we suppose specifically that $(X_{i1}, \ldots, X_{in_i})$ is a random sample of size n_i from the i-th Bernoulli population with unknown success probability p_i $(i = 1, \ldots, k)$. Furthermore, X_{ij}'s are assumed to be independent. Under same sample sizes of $n_1 = \ldots = n_k$, Bartholomew (1959) and Shi (1991) constructed tests for null hypothesis $H_0 : p_1 = \ldots = p_k$ versus the ordered alternative $H^A : p_1 \le p_2 \le \ldots \le p_k$ with at least one strict inequality. Even if the null hypothesis H_0 is rejected by using their procedures, we only get the conclusion of $p_1 < p_k$, which simply represents the presence of monotonicity, indicating many possible differential patterns among the groups of interest. Multiple comparison procedures can detect more specific differences among the groups that are of interest.

© The Author(s), under exclusive license to Springer Nature Singapore Pte Ltd. 2022　　61
T. Shiraishi, *Multiple Comparisons for Bernoulli Data,*
JSS Research Series in Statistics,
https://doi.org/10.1007/978-981-19-2708-9_6

Such procedures are more informative and thus more useful for clinical trials and experiments in agriculture or other fields. We consider multiple comparison procedures in k-sample models. For specified i, i' such that $1 \leq i < i' \leq k$, if we are interested in testing

the null hypothesis $H_{(i,i')} : p_i = p_{i'}$ versus the alternative $H^{A*}_{(i,i')} : p_i < p_{i'}$, (6.2)

we can use the one-sided two-sample z-test. In this chapter, we consider test procedures for all-pairwise comparisons of $\{$the null hypothesis $H_{(i,i')}$ versus the alternative $H^{A*}_{(i,i')} \mid (i, i') \in \mathcal{U}_k\}$, where

$$\mathcal{U}_k = \{(i, i') \mid 1 \leq i < i' \leq k\}.$$

Under the usual normality, simple order restrictions of means and equality of sample sizes, Hayter (1990) proposed single-step procedures as multiple comparison tests of level α in the homoscedastic k-sample model. Shiraishi (2014a) and Shiraishi et al. (2019) show that (i) they are more powerful than the single-step procedures of Hayter (1990), and (ii) confidence regions induced by the multi-step procedures are equivalent to simultaneous confidence intervals.

We state the Hayter-type procedure similar to the normal theory of all-pairwise comparisons of $\{$the null hypothesis $H_{(i,i')}$ versus the alternative $H^A_{(i,i')} \mid (i, i') \in \mathcal{U}_k\}$. Furthermore, we discuss closed testing procedures which are based on statistics having asymptotically a $\bar{\chi}^2$-distribution, which appeared in Chernoff (1954).

Throughout this chapter, we suppose that the assumption of (A1) stated in Sect. 3.1 is satisfied.

Procedures and theory stated in this chapter are used in hybrid serial gatekeeping procedures for all-pairwise comparisons of Chap. 8.

6.2 $\bar{\chi}^2$-Test

For k-sample models with Bernoulli responses of the previous section, $X_i = \sum_{j=1}^{n_i} X_{ij}$ has the binomial distribution with parameters n_i and p_i, and estimators of p_i's are given by $\hat{p}_i = X_i/n_i$ or $(X_i + 0.5)/(n_i + 1)$ $(i = 1, \ldots, k)$. We put $n := \sum_{i=1}^k n_i$.

Let us put $\hat{v}_i := 2 \arcsin\left(\sqrt{\hat{p}_i}\right)$ and $v_i = 2 \arcsin\left(\sqrt{p_i}\right)$. Then using a central limit theorem and Slutsky's theorem, under (A1), we get

$$\sqrt{n}\left(\hat{v}_i - v_i\right) \xrightarrow{\mathcal{L}} Y_i \sim N\left(0, \frac{1}{\lambda_i}\right), \tag{6.3}$$

where $\xrightarrow{\mathcal{L}}$ denotes convergence in law and $Y \sim N(0, \sigma^2)$ denotes that Y is distributed according to $N(0, \sigma^2)$. $T_{i'i}$ of (3.7) is expressed as

$$T_{i'i} = \frac{\hat{v}_{i'} - \hat{v}_i}{\sqrt{\frac{1}{n_i} + \frac{1}{n_{i'}}}} \quad (i < i').$$

When the simple order restrictions of (6.1) is satisfied, we consider the null hypothesis H_0 versus the alternative H^A : $p_1 \leq p_2 \leq \ldots \leq p_k$ with at least one strict inequality, which is equivalent to H_0 : $p_1 = p_k$ versus H^A : $p_1 < p_k$. We define $\{\hat{v}_i^* \mid i = 1, \ldots, k\}$ by $\{u_i \mid i = 1, \ldots, k\}$ which minimize $\sum_{i=1}^{k} \lambda_{ni} \left(u_i - \hat{v}_i\right)^2$ under simple order restrictions $u_1 \leq u_2 \leq \ldots \leq u_k$, i.e.,

$$\sum_{i=1}^{k} \lambda_{ni} \left(\hat{v}_i^* - \hat{v}_i\right)^2 = \min_{u_1 \leq \ldots \leq u_k} \sum_{i=1}^{k} \lambda_{ni} \left(u_i - \hat{v}_i\right)^2,$$

where $\lambda_{ni} := n_i/n$ $(1 \leq i \leq k)$. $\hat{v}_1^*, \ldots, \hat{v}_k^*$ are computed by using the pool-adjacent-violators algorithm stated in Robertson et al. (1988) and

$$\hat{v}_i^* = \max_{1 \leq a \leq i} \min_{i \leq b \leq k} \frac{\sum_{j=a}^{b} \lambda_{nj} \hat{v}_j}{\sum_{j=a}^{b} \lambda_{nj}} = \max_{1 \leq a \leq i} \min_{i \leq b \leq k} \frac{\sum_{j=a}^{b} n_j \hat{v}_j}{\sum_{j=a}^{b} n_j}$$

holds. We put

$$\bar{\chi}_k^2 := \sum_{i=1}^{k} n_i \left(\hat{v}_i^* - \sum_{j=1}^{k} \lambda_{nj} \hat{v}_j\right)^2.$$

We define $\tilde{v}_1^*, \ldots, \tilde{v}_k^*$ by

$$\sum_{i=1}^{k} \lambda_i \left(\tilde{v}_i^* - Y_i\right)^2 = \min_{u_1 \leq \ldots \leq u_k} \sum_{i=1}^{k} \lambda_i (u_i - Y_i)^2,$$

where Y_i is defined in (6.3). Let $P(L, k; \lambda)$ be the probability that $\tilde{v}_1^*, \ldots, \tilde{v}_k^*$ takes exactly L distinct values, where $\lambda := (\lambda_1, \ldots, \lambda_k)$. Then, for positive constant c, $P(L, k; c\lambda) = P(L, k; \lambda)$ holds. Furthermore, by using (6.3) and Theorem 2.3.1 of Robertson et al. (1988), we get, under (A1),

$$\lim_{n \to \infty} P_0(\bar{\chi}_k^2 \geq t) = \sum_{L=2}^{k} P(L, k; \lambda) P\left(\chi_{L-1}^2 \geq t\right) \quad (t > 0), \tag{6.4}$$

where $P_0(\cdot)$ denotes the probability measure under H_0 and χ_{L-1}^2 is a chi-square variable with $L - 1$ degrees of freedom. The recurrence formula of computing $P(L, k; \lambda)$ is written in Robertson et al. (1988). We shall state the recurrence formula along the above notations. Hayter and Liu (1996) showed that the value of

$$P(k, k; \lambda) = P(Y_1 < Y_2 < \ldots < Y_k) \tag{6.5}$$

can be derived by the recurrence of one-dimensional computational integration. Let $I_1^d, I_2^d, \ldots, I_L^d$ be a partition of $\{1, 2, \ldots, k\}$ satisfying the following property (P1).

(P1) Each I_s^d is a nonempty set composed of consecutive integers or an integer. When $L \geq 2$, the maximum value of the elements of I_i^d is less than the minimum value of I_{i+1}^d for any integer i such that $1 \leq i \leq L - 1$.

Then Theorem 2.4.1 of Robertson et al. (1988) gives, for $L = 2, \ldots, k - 1$,

$$P(L, k; \lambda) = \sum_{\{I_1^d, I_2^d, \ldots, I_L^d\}} P\left(L, L; \Lambda(I_1^d), \Lambda(I_2^d), \ldots, \Lambda(I_L^d)\right) \cdot \prod_{s=1}^{L} P(1, \#(I_s^d); \lambda(I_s^d)),$$
$$\tag{6.6}$$

where $\#(I_s^d)$ denotes the number of elements of I_s^d, $\Lambda(I_s^d) = \sum_{i \in I_s^d} \lambda_i$, $\lambda(I_s^d) = (\lambda_i, \lambda_{i+1}, \ldots, \lambda_j)$ for $I_s^d = \{i, i+1, \ldots, j\}$, and $\sum_{\{I_1^d, I_2^d, \ldots, I_L^d\}}$ denotes the sum over all partitions of $\{1, 2, \ldots, k\}$ satisfying (P1). $\#(I_s^d)$ of (6.6) is less than or equal to $k - 1$. Furthermore, we get

$$P(1, k; \lambda) = 1 - \sum_{L=2}^{k} P(L, k : \lambda)$$

and

$$P(1, 1; \lambda_i) = 1 \quad (1 \leq i \leq k), \tag{6.7}$$

$$P(1, 2; \lambda_i, \lambda_j) = P(2, 2; \lambda_i, \lambda_j) = \frac{1}{2} \quad (1 \leq i < j \leq k). \tag{6.8}$$

Since $P(L, k; \lambda)$ depends on L and k for

$$\lambda_1 = \ldots = \lambda_k = 1/k, \tag{6.9}$$

$P(L, k; \lambda)$ is abbreviated as $P(L, k)$ under (6.9). Barlow et al. (1972) give the following recurrence formula.

$$P(1, k) = \frac{1}{k},$$

$$P(L, k) = \frac{1}{k}\{(k - 1)P(L, k - 1) + P(L - 1, k - 1)\} \quad (2 \leq L \leq k - 1),$$

$$P(k, k) = \frac{1}{k!}.$$

For given α such that $0 < \alpha < 1$, we give the following equation of t.

$$\sum_{L=2}^{k} P(L,k;\lambda)P\left(\chi_{L-1}^2 \geq t\right) = \alpha.$$

We denote a solution of this equation by $\bar{c}^2(k,\lambda;\alpha)$. Hence, from (6.4), we can reject H_0 when the value of $\bar{\chi}_k^2$ is larger than $\bar{c}^2(k,\lambda;\alpha)$. The values of $\bar{c}^2(k,\lambda;\alpha)$ for the condition (6.9) are stated in Table A.3 of Barlow et al. (1972).

6.3 Single-Step Procedures

Under the ordered restriction (6.1), we consider test procedures for all-pairwise comparisons of

{the null hypothesis $H_{(i,i')} : p_i = p_{i'}$ versus the alternative $H_{(i,i')}^A : p_i < p_{i'} | (i,i') \in \mathscr{U}_k$}.

We add the assumption (A2) of same sample sizes.

(A2) $\qquad n_1 = n_2 = \ldots = n_k = n_0.$
Then $T_{i'i}^{(r)}$ is given by

$$T_{i'i} = \sqrt{2n_0} \left\{ \arcsin\left(\sqrt{\hat{p}_{i'}}\right) - \arcsin\left(\sqrt{\hat{p}_i}\right) \right\}.$$

We put

$$D_1(t|k) = P\left(\max_{1 \leq i < i' \leq k} \frac{Z_{i'} - Z_i}{\sqrt{2}} \leq t\right), \qquad (6.10)$$

where $Z_i \sim N(0,1)$ and $Z_1, \ldots, Z_k$ are independent. Shiraishi (2014b) gives

$$\lim_{n\to\infty} P_0\left(\max_{1 \leq i < i' \leq k} T_{i'i} \leq t\right) = D_1(t|k). \qquad (6.11)$$

From Hayter and Liu (1996), we can get the value of $D_1(t|k)$ by using the recurrence relation

$$h_1(t,y) = \Phi(\sqrt{2}\cdot t + y),$$

$$h_r(t,y) = \int_{-\infty}^{y} h_{r-1}(t,y)\varphi(y)dy + h_{r-1}(t,y)\{\Phi(\sqrt{2}\cdot t + y) - \Phi(y)\} \ (2 \leq r \leq k-1),$$

$$D_1(t|k) = \int_{-\infty}^{\infty} h_{k-1}(t,y)\varphi(y)dy, \qquad (6.12)$$

where $\varphi(y)$ denotes a standard normal density function. We denote the solution of $D_1(t|k) = 1 - \alpha$ by $d_1(k;\alpha)$, i.e., $D_1(d_1(k;\alpha)|k) = 1 - \alpha$. Then, from (6.11), Shiraishi (2014b) proposed the following procedures similar to the normal theory of Hayter (1990).

Table 6.1 The values of $d_1(k; \alpha)$ for $\alpha = 0.05, \ 0.01$ and $k = 3(1)10$

$100\alpha\% \setminus k$	3	4	5	6	7	8	9	10
5%	2.081	2.329	2.502	2.634	2.740	2.828	2.904	2.969
1%	2.693	2.907	3.058	3.173	3.266	3.345	3.412	3.470

[6.1] Hayter-Type Simultaneous Intervals

The asymptotic $100(1 - \alpha)\%$ simultaneous confidence intervals for $\{\arcsin(\sqrt{p_{i'}}) - \arcsin(\sqrt{p_i}) \mid (i, i') \in \mathscr{U}_k\}$ are given by

$$\arcsin(\sqrt{\hat{p}_{i'}}) - \arcsin(\sqrt{\hat{p}_i}) - \frac{d_1(k; \alpha)}{\sqrt{2n_0}} < \arcsin(\sqrt{p_{i'}}) - \arcsin(\sqrt{p_i}) < +\infty \quad ((i, i') \in \mathscr{U}_k).$$

$$(6.13)$$

[6.2] Single-Step Tests

Asymptotic simultaneous tests of level α for {the null hypothesis $H_{(i,i')}$ versus the alternative $H^A_{(i,i')} \mid (i, i') \in \mathscr{U}_k$} consist in rejecting $H_{(i,i')}$ for $(i, i') \in \mathscr{U}_k$ such that $T_{i'i} > d_1(k; \alpha)$.

The values of $d_1(k; \alpha)$ for $\alpha = 0.05, 0.01$ and $k = 3(6.1)10$ are provided in Table 6.1.

6.4 Closed Testing Procedures

Assume that the ordered restrictions (6.1) are satisfied. Then we put

$$\mathscr{H}_3 := \{H_{(i,i')} \mid (i, i') \in \mathscr{U}_k\}.$$

The closure of $\mathscr{H}_3$ is given by

$$\overline{\mathscr{H}}_3 = \left\{ \bigwedge_{v \in V} H_v \ \middle| \ \emptyset \subsetneq V \subset \mathscr{U}_k \right\},$$

where $\bigwedge$ denotes the conjunction symbol (Refer to Enderton (2001)). Then, we get

$$\bigwedge_{v \in V} H_v : \text{for any } (i, i') \in V, \ p_i = p_{i'}.$$

$$(6.14)$$

Let $I_1, \ldots, I_J$ be disjoint sets satisfying the following property (P2).

(P2) There exist integers $\ell_1, \ldots, \ell_J \geq 2$ and integers $0 \leq s_1 < \ldots < s_J < k$ such that

$$I_j = \{s_j + 1, s_j + 2, \ldots s_j + \ell_j\} \ (j = 1, \ldots, J),$$

$$s_j + \ell_j \le s_{j+1} \ (j = 1, \ldots, J - 1) \text{ and } s_J \le k.$$

We define the null hypothesis $H^O(I_1, \ldots, I_J)$ by

$$H^O(I_1, \ldots, I_J) : \text{for any } j \text{ such that } 1 \le j \le J \text{ and for any } i, i' \in I_j,$$
$$p_i = p_{i'} \text{ holds.} \tag{6.15}$$

The elements of I_j are consecutive integers and $\#(I_j) \ge 2$. From (6.14) and (6.15), for any nonempty $V \subset \mathcal{U}_k$, there exist an integer J and some subsets $I_1, \ldots, I_J \subset \{1, \ldots, k\}$ satisfying (P2) such that

$$\bigwedge_{v \in V} H_v = H^O(I_1, \ldots, I_J). \tag{6.16}$$

Furthermore, $H^O(I_1, \ldots, I_J)$ is expressed as

$$H^O(I_1, \ldots, I_J) : \ p_{s_j+1} = p_{s_j+2} = \ldots = p_{s_j+\ell_j} \ (j = 1, \ldots, J). \tag{6.17}$$

For $H^O(I_1, \ldots, I_J)$ of (6.16), we set

$$M := M(I_1, \ldots, I_J) = \sum_{j=1}^{J} \ell_j, \ \ell_j = \#(I_j). \tag{6.18}$$

For $\ell = \ell_1, \ldots, \ell_J$, we define $\alpha(M, \ell)$ by

$$\alpha(M, \ell) = 1 - (1 - \alpha)^{\ell/M}.$$

For ℓ such that $2 \le \ell \le k$, we put

$$D_1(t|\ell) := P\left(\max_{1 \le i < i' \le \ell} \frac{Z_{i'} - Z_i}{\sqrt{2}} \le t\right), \tag{6.19}$$

where Z_i's are random variables used in (6.10). $D_1(d_1(\ell; \alpha)|\ell) = 1 - \alpha$ holds.
    Then, we propose a stepwise procedure.

[6.3] Stepwise Procedure Based on One-Sided Z-Test Statistics

The condition (A2) is assumed. We put

$$T^O(I_j) := \max_{s_j+1 \le i < i' \le s_j+\ell_j} T_{i'i} \ (j = 1, \ldots, J).$$

(a) $J \geq 2$

Whenever $d_1\left(\ell_j; \alpha(M, \ell_j)\right) < T^O(I_j)$ holds for an integer j such that $1 \leq j \leq J$, we reject the hypothesis $\bigwedge_{\nu \in V} H_\nu$.

(b) $J = 1$ $(M = \ell_1)$

Whenever $d_1(M; \alpha) < T^O(I_1)$, we reject the hypothesis $\bigwedge_{\nu \in V} H_\nu$.

By using the methods of (a) and (b), when $\bigwedge_{\nu \in V} H_\nu$ is rejected for any V such that $(i, i') \in V \subset \mathcal{U}_k$, the null hypothesis $H_{(i,i')}$ is rejected as a multiple comparison test. Then, this procedure also becomes a closed test.

For $\alpha = 0.05,\ 0.01$, we give the values of $d_1(\ell; \alpha(M, \ell))$ in Tables 6.2 and 6.3, respectively. We limited attention to $2 \leq M \leq 10$. $\ell = M - 1$ is not used in the procedure [6.3]. When $\ell = M = k$ is satisfied, $d_1(\ell; \alpha(M, \ell)) = d_1(k; \alpha)$ holds.

Theorem 6.1 *The stepwise procedure of [6.3] is an asymptotic multiple comparison test of level α.*

Proof It is trivial to verify that the level of the test procedure of (b) is α. We show that the level of the test procedure of (a) is α. Furthermore, we suppose without any loss of generality that H_0 is true. Since $T^O(I_1), \ldots, T^O(I_J)$ are independent, we get

$$\lim_{n \to \infty} P_0\left(T^O(I_j) \leqq d_1\left(\ell_j; \alpha(M, \ell_j)\right)\right),\ j = 1, \ldots, J$$

$$= \prod_{j=1}^{J}\left\{\lim_{n \to \infty} P_0\left(T^O(I_j) \leqq d_1\left(\ell_j; \alpha(M, \ell_j)\right)\right)\right\}$$

$$= \prod_{j=1}^{J}\{1 - \alpha(M, \ell_j)\}$$

$$= 1 - \alpha. \tag{6.20}$$

From (6.20), we have

$$\lim_{n \to \infty} P_0\left(\text{There exists } j \text{ such that } T^O(I_j) > d_1\left(\ell_j; \alpha(M, \ell_j)\right)\right)$$

$$= 1 - \lim_{n \to \infty} P_0\left(T^O(I_j) \leqq d_1\left(\ell_j; \alpha(M, \ell_j)\right)\right),\ j = 1, \ldots, J$$

$$= \alpha.$$

Therefore, the level of the test procedure of (a) for the null hypothesis $\bigwedge_{\nu \in V} H_\nu$ is asymptotically α. Hence, the assertion of the theorem is proved.   □

Table 6.2 The values of $d_1 (\ell; \alpha(M, \ell))$ for $\alpha = 0.05$ and $M = 2(1)10$

$M \setminus \ell$	2	3	4	5	6	7	8	9	10
10	2.319	2.545	2.668	2.751	2.814	2.864	2.905	◊	2.969
9	2.279	2.507	2.631	2.715	2.778	2.828	◊	2.904	
8	2.234	2.464	2.589	2.674	2.737	◊	2.828		
7	2.182	2.415	2.541	2.626	◊	2.740			
6	2.121	2.357	2.484	◊	2.634				
5	2.047	2.287	◊	2.502					
4	1.955	◊	2.329						
3	◊	2.081							
2	1.645								

The places of ◊ are not used in the procedure [6.3]

Table 6.3 The values of $d_1 (\ell; \alpha(M, \ell))$ for $\alpha = 0.01$ and $M = 2(1)10$

$M \setminus \ell$	2	3	4	5	6	7	8	9	10
10	2.877	3.078	3.190	3.266	3.324	3.370	3.409	◊	3.470
9	2.844	3.046	3.158	3.235	3.293	3.340	◊	3.412	
8	2.806	3.010	3.123	3.200	3.259	◊	3.345		
7	2.763	2.969	3.083	3.161	◊	3.266			
6	2.712	2.920	3.035	◊	3.173				
5	2.651	2.862	◊	3.058					
4	2.575	◊	2.907						
3	◊	2.693							
2	2.326								

From (6.16), we find

$$\overline{\mathscr{H}}_3 = \left\{ H^O(I_1, \ldots, I_J) \;\middle|\; \text{There exists } J \text{ such that } \bigcup_{j=1}^{J} I_j \subset \{1, \ldots, k\}, \right.$$

$$I_j \text{ satisfies (P2)}, \#(I_j) \geq 2 \ (1 \leq j \leq J),$$

$$\left. \text{and } I_j \cap I_{j'} = \emptyset \ (1 \leq j < j' \leq J) \text{ for } J \geq 2 \right\}.$$

For $(i, i') \in \mathscr{U}_k$, we put

$$\overline{\mathscr{H}}_{3(i,i')} := \left\{ H^O(I_1, \ldots, I_J) \in \overline{\mathscr{H}}_3 \;\middle|\; \text{There exists } j \text{ such that satisfies } 1 \leq j \leq J \text{ and } \{i, i'\} \subset I_j \right\}.$$

Then we get

$$\overline{\mathscr{H}}_3 = \bigcup_{(i,i') \in \mathscr{U}_k} \overline{\mathscr{H}}_{3(i,i')}, \text{ and } H_{(i,i')}, \; H_0 \in \overline{\mathscr{H}}_{3(i,i')}.$$

Furthermore, for $1 \leq i_1 \leq i_2 < i_2' \leq i_1' \leq k$,

$$\overline{\mathcal{H}}_{3(i_1, i_1')} \subset \overline{\mathcal{H}}_{3(i_2, i_2')} \tag{6.21}$$

holds. $\overline{\mathcal{H}}_{3(i,i')}$ is the family of $H^O(I_1, \ldots, I_J)$'s tested to reject specified null hypothesis $H_{(i,i')}$.

We consider the example of $k = 4$. $\overline{\mathcal{H}}_{3(i,i')}$'s are given by

$$\overline{\mathcal{H}}_{3(1,2)} = \{H^O(\{1,2,3,4\}),\ H^O(\{1,2\},\{3,4\}),\ H^O(\{1,2,3\}),\ H^O(\{1,2\})\},$$
$$\overline{\mathcal{H}}_{3(1,3)} = \{H^O(\{1,2,3,4\}),\ H^O(\{1,2,3\})\},$$
$$\overline{\mathcal{H}}_{3(1,4)} = \{H^O(\{1,2,3,4\})\},$$
$$\overline{\mathcal{H}}_{3(2,3)} = \{H^O(\{1,2,3,4\}),\ H^O(\{1,2,3\}),\ H^O(\{2,3,4\}),\ H^O(\{2,3\})\},$$
$$\overline{\mathcal{H}}_{3(2,4)} = \{H^O(\{1,2,3,4\}),\ H^O(\{2,3,4\})\},$$
$$\overline{\mathcal{H}}_{3(3,4)} = \{H^O(\{1,2,3,4\}),\ H^O(\{1,2\},\{3,4\}),\ H^O(\{2,3,4\}),\ H^O(\{3,4\})\}.$$

Hence, by using the multi-step procedure [6.3] as a multiple test procedure, $H^O(I_1, \ldots, I_J)$'s tested to reject specified null hypothesis $H_{(1,2)}$ are as follows.

$H^O(\{1,2,3,4\})$: $p_1 = p_2 = p_3 = p_4$; $J = 1$, $s_1 = 0$, $\ell_1 = 4$

$H^O(\{1,2\},\{3,4\})$: $p_1 = p_2$, $p_3 = p_4$; $J = 2$, $s_1 = 0$, $\ell_1 = 2$, $s_2 = 2$, $\ell_2 = 2$

$H^O(\{1,2,3\})$: $p_1 = p_2 = p_3$; $J = 1$, $s_1 = 0$, $\ell_1 = 3$

$H^O(\{1,2\}) = H_{(1,2)}$: $p_1 = p_2$; $J = 1$, $s_1 = 0$, $\ell_1 = 2$.

From Table 6.2, the null hypothesis $H_{(1,2)}$ is rejected as the closed test procedures of level 0.05 whenever the following inequalities (6.22)–(6.25) are satisfied.

$$T^O(\{1,2,3,4\}) = \max_{1 \leq i < i' \leq 4} T_{i'i} \geq 2.329 \tag{6.22}$$

$$T^O(\{1,2\},\{3,4\}) = \max\{T_{21},\ T_{43}\} \geq 1.955 \tag{6.23}$$

$$T^O(\{1,2,3\}) = \max_{1 \leq i < i' \leq 3} T_{i'i} \geq 2.081 \tag{6.24}$$

$$T_{21} \geq 1.645. \tag{6.25}$$

For $\alpha = 0.05$, 0.01 and $4 \leq k \leq 10$, from Tables 6.2 and 6.3, we find

$$d_1(\ell; \alpha(M, \ell)) < d_1(k; \alpha(k, k)) = d_1(k; \alpha) \tag{6.26}$$

for ℓ such that $2 \leq \ell < M \leq k$. By numerical calculation, we verify that (6.26) holds for $\alpha = 0.05$, 0.01 and $3 \leq k \leq 10$. From the construction of the closed testing procedure [6.3] and the relation of (6.26), we get the following (i) and (ii). (i) The procedure [6.3] of level α rejects $H_{(i,i')}$ that is rejected by the single-step simultaneous test [6.2] of level α. (ii) The single-step simultaneous test [6.2] of level α does not always reject $H_{(i,i')}$ that is rejected by the procedure [6.3] of level α. Hence, for $\alpha = 0.05$, 0.01 and $3 \le k \le 10$, the closed testing procedure [6.3] is more powerful than the single-step simultaneous test [6.2].

We get Theorem 6.2 as in the proof of Theorem 3.3.

Theorem 6.2 *Let $A_{(i,i')}$ be the event that $H_{(i,i')}$ is rejected by the procedure [6.3] as a multiple comparison of level α $((i, i') \in \mathcal{U}_k)$. Suppose that*

$$d_1 \left(\ell; \alpha(M, \ell) \right) < d_1(k; \alpha) \tag{6.27}$$

is satisfied for any M such that $4 \le M \le k$ and any integer ℓ such that $2 \le \ell \le M - 2$, where M is defined by (6.18). Then the following relations hold.

$$P \left(\bigcup_{(i,i') \in \mathcal{U}_k} A_{(i,i')} \right) = P \left(\max_{1 \le i < i' \le k} T_{i'i} > d_1(k; \alpha) \right)$$

$$P \left(A_{(i,i')} \right) \ge P \left(T_{i'i} > d_1(k; \alpha) \right) \quad ((i, i') \in \mathcal{U}_k). \qquad \square$$

Next we do not assume the condition of (A2), Sample sizes may be uneven. For $j = 1, \ldots, J$, we define $(\hat{v}^*_{s_j+1}(I_j), \ldots, \hat{v}^*_{s_j+\ell_j}(I_j))$ by $(u_{s_j+1}, \ldots, u_{s_j+\ell_j})$ which minimize $\sum_{i \in I_j} \lambda_{ni} \left(u_i - \hat{v}_i \right)^2$ under simple order restrictions $u_{s_j+1} \le u_{s_j+2} \le \ldots \le u_{s_j+\ell_j}$, i.e.,

$$\sum_{i \in I_j} \lambda_{ni} \left(\hat{v}^*_i(I_j) - \hat{v}_i \right)^2 = \min_{u_{s_j+1} \le \ldots \le u_{s_j+\ell_j}} \sum_{i \in I_j} \lambda_{ni} \left(u_i - \hat{v}_i \right)^2,$$

where I_j, s_j, and ℓ_j are defined in (P2).

[6.4] Stepwise Procedure Based on $\bar{\chi}^2$ Statistics
Let us put

$$\bar{\chi}^2_{\ell_j}(I_j) := \sum_{i \in I_j} n_i \left(\hat{v}^*_i(I_j) - \sum_{i \in I_j} \left(\frac{n_i}{n(I_j)} \right) \hat{v}_i \right)^2 \quad (j = 1, \ldots, J),$$

where $n(I_j) = \sum_{i \in I_j} n_i$.

From the discussion similar to (6.4), we have

$$\lim_{n \to \infty} P_0(\bar{\chi}^2_{\ell_j}(I_j) \ge t) = \sum_{L=2}^{\ell_j} P(L, \ell_j; \lambda(I_j)) P \left(\chi^2_{L-1} \ge t \right), \quad (t > 0)$$

where $\lambda(I_j) := (\lambda_{s_j+1}, \lambda_{s_j+2}, \ldots, \lambda_{s_j+\ell_j})$. For a given β such that $0 < \beta < 1$, we put

Table 6.4 Critical values $\bar{c}^2(\ell, \alpha(M, \ell))$ for the powerful stepwise procedure

(a) $\alpha = 0.05$

$M \setminus \ell$	2	3	4	5	6	7	8	9	10
10	5.376	6.022	6.302	6.445	6.521	6.558	6.572	◊	6.560
9	5.194	5.825	6.095	6.231	6.301	6.334	◊	6.339	
8	4.991	5.606	5.865	5.993	6.056	◊	6.088		
7	4.762	5.359	5.606	5.724	◊	5.800			
6	4.499	5.075	5.307	◊	5.460				
5	4.192	4.740	◊	5.049					
4	3.820	◊	4.528						
3	◊	3.820							
2	2.706								

The places of ◊ are not used in the procedure [6.4].

(b) $\alpha = 0.01$

$M \setminus \ell$	2	3	4	5	6	7	8	9	10
10	8.277	9.118	9.532	9.779	9.939	10.048	10.124	◊	10.216
9	8.086	8.916	9.322	9.562	9.717	9.822	◊	9.945	
8	7.873	8.690	9.087	9.320	9.470	◊	9.638		
7	7.632	8.434	8.821	9.046	◊	9.284			
6	7.355	8.139	8.514	◊	8.865				
5	7.028	7.792	◊	8.356					
4	6.630	◊	7.709						
3	◊	6.823							
2	5.412								

$\bar{c}^2\left(\ell_j, \lambda(I_j); \beta\right) := $ a solution of t satisfying the equation

$$\sum_{L=2}^{\ell_j} P(L, \ell_j; \lambda(I_j)) P\left(\chi_{L-1}^2 \geq t\right) = \beta.$$

(a) $J \geq 2$
Whenever $\bar{c}^2\left(\ell_j, \lambda(I_j); \alpha(M, \ell_j)\right) < \bar{\chi}_{\ell_j}^2(I_j)$ holds for an integer j such that $1 \leq j \leq J$, we reject the hypothesis $\bigwedge_{v \in V} H_v$.
(b) $J = 1$ ($M = \ell_1$)
Whenever $\bar{c}^2\left(\ell_1, \lambda(I_1); \alpha\right) < \bar{\chi}_{\ell_1}^2(I_1)$, we reject the hypothesis $\bigwedge_{v \in V} H_v$.

By using the methods of (a) and (b), when $\bigwedge_{v \in V} H_v$ is rejected for any V such that $(i, i') \in V \subset \mathcal{U}_k$, the null hypothesis $H_{(i,i')}$ is rejected as a multiple comparison test.

By the proof similar to the proof of Theorem 6.1, we get Theorem 6.3.

Theorem 6.3 *Under (A1), the level for test procedure [6.4] is asymptotically α as a multiple comparison test.* ☐

When the condition (A2) is satisfied, $\bar{c}^2(\ell, \lambda(I); \alpha(M, \ell))$ does not depend on $\lambda(I)$ for $(\ell, I) = (\ell_1, I_1), \ldots, (\ell_J, I_J)$. Hence, under (A2), we rewrite $\bar{c}_\ell^2(\lambda(I); \alpha(M, \ell))$ as $\bar{c}_\ell^2(\alpha(M, \ell))$ shortly.

For $\alpha = 0.05, 0.01$, we give the values of $\bar{c}_\ell^2(\alpha(M, \ell))$ in Table 6.4.

We limited attention to $2 \le M \le 10$. The values of $\bar{c}^2(\ell, \alpha(M, \ell))$ for $\ell = M - 1$ are not used. We consider $k = 4$. By the same method as multi-step procedure [6.3], to reject $H_{(1,2)}$ as a multiple test, the rejection of the four null hypotheses in $\overline{\mathcal{H}}_{3(1,2)}$ is required. Therefore, if the following conditions (i)–(iv) are satisfied, $H_{(1,2)}$ is rejected as a multiple test of level α based on the procedure [6.4].

(i) $\bar{\chi}_4^2(\{1, 2, 3, 4\}) > \bar{c}^2(4, n_1/n, n_2/n, n_3/n, n_4/n, ; \alpha)$.

(ii) $\bar{\chi}_2^2(\{1, 2\}) > \bar{c}^2(2, n_1/n, n_2/n, ; \alpha(4, 2))$ or $\bar{\chi}_2^2(\{3, 4\}) > \bar{c}^2(2, n_3/n, n_4/n, ; \alpha(4, 2))$.

(iii) $\bar{\chi}_3^2(\{1, 2, 3\}) > \bar{c}^2(3, n_1/n, n_2/n, n_3/n, ; \alpha)$.

(iv) $\bar{\chi}_2^2(\{1, 2\}) > \bar{c}^2(2, n_1/n, n_2/n, ; \alpha)$.

References

Agresti A, Coull BA (1996) Order-restricted tests for stratified comparisons of binomial proportions. Biometrics 52:1103–1111

Barlow RE, Bartholomew DJ, Bremner JM, Brunk HD (1972) Statistical inference under order restrictions. Wiley, London

Bartholomew DJ (1959) A test of homogeneity for ordered alternatives. Biometrika 46:36–48

Chernoff H (1954) On the distribution of the likelihood ratio. Ann Math Statist 25:573–578

Enderton HB (2001) A mathematical introduction to logic, 2nd edn. Academic Press

Hayter AJ (1990) A one-sided studentized range test for testing against a simple ordered alternative. J Amer Statist Assoc 85:778–785

Hayter AJ, Liu W (1996) On the exact calculation of the one-sided studentized range test. Computat stat data Anal 22:17–25

Robertson T, Wright FT, Dykstra RL (1988) Order restricted statistical inference. Wiley, New York

Shi NZ (1991) A test of homogeneity of odds ratios against order restrictions. J Amer Statist Assoc 86:154–158

Shiraishi T (2014) Closed testing procedures in multi-sample models under a simple ordered restriction. J Japan Statist Soc 43:215–245 (in Japanese)

Shiraishi T (2014) Multiple comparison procedures for a simple ordered restriction in multi-sample models with bernoulli responses. Japanese Soc Appl Statist 43:1–22 (in Japanese)

Shiraishi T, Sugiura H, Matsuda S (2019) Pairwise multiple comparisons-theory and computation. Springer

Chapter 7
Comparisons with a Control and Successive Comparisons Under Simple Order Restrictions

Abstract Multiple comparison procedures for ordered means are proposed by Williams (1971, 1972) and Lee and Spurrier (1995) in k normal populations. First, we consider multiple comparison procedures for the differences among proportions in k binomial populations under simple order restrictions. We may discuss Williams-type test procedures based on arcsine transformation under the equality of sample sizes. Furthermore, we may propose a closed testing procedure that is superior to the Hayter-type test procedure. Also, we propose closed testing procedures based on statistics having asymptotically a $\bar{\chi}^2$-distribution which appeared in Chernoff (1954). Next, we consider multiple comparison procedures for successive comparisons between ordered proportions. We may discuss Lee-Spurrier-type single-step procedures. We may propose a closed testing procedure that is superior to the Lee-Spurrier-type test procedure.

7.1 Introduction

In many applications of k-sample models for comparing proportions in clinical trials or experimental studies, individuals are classified as two possible outcomes, "success" and "failure". Let $p_1, \ldots, p_k$ correspond to the probabilities that individuals at each of k levels of control or treatment possess "success". For this setting, Agresti and Coull (1996) assumed k-sample Bernoulli responses models with the simple order restrictions

$$p_1 \leq p_2 \leq \ldots \leq p_k. \tag{7.1}$$

For the k-sample models, we suppose specifically that $(X_{i1}, \ldots, X_{in_i})$ is a random sample of size n_i from the i-th Bernoulli population with unknown success probability p_i $(i = 1, \ldots, k)$. Furthermore, X_{ij}'s are assumed to be independent.

We consider multiple comparison procedures in k-sample models with the simple order restrictions of (7.1). Under the assumption of

$$n_2 = \ldots = n_k, \tag{A3}$$

we may propose the Williams-type procedure based on arcsine transformation for comparisons with a control of $\{$the null hypothesis $H_i : p_i = p_1$ versus the alternative $H_i^{A+} : p_i > p_1 | i \in \mathscr{I}_{2,k}\}$, where

$$\mathscr{I}_{2,k} := \{i \mid 2 \leq i \leq k\}. \tag{7.2}$$

Furthermore, we may propose a closed testing procedure based on statistics having asymptotically a $\bar{\chi}^2$-distribution, which appeared in Chernoff (1954). In the theory of this closed testing procedure, the condition (A3) is not needed.

Next, we may propose the Lee-Spurrier-type single-step test procedure for successive comparisons of $\{$the null hypothesis $H_{(i,i+1)} : p_i = p_{i+1}$ versus the alternative $H_{(i,i+1)}^A : p_i < p_{i+1} | i \in \mathscr{I}_{1,k-1}\}$, where

$$\mathscr{I}_{1,k-1} := \{i \mid 1 \leq i \leq k - 1\}. \tag{7.3}$$

We propose closed testing procedures as multiple comparison tests that is superior to the Lee-Spurrier-type single-step test procedure.

Throughout this chapter, we suppose that the assumption of (A1) stated in Sect. 3.1 is satisfied.

Procedures and theory stated in this chapter are used in hybrid serial gatekeeping procedures for multiple comparisons with a control of Chap. 9.

7.2   Multiple Comparison Tests with a Control

We assume that the ordered restriction (7.1) is satisfied. The first treatment is regarded as a control with which the remaining $k - 1$ treatments are to be compared. In one comparison, we test the null hypothesis $H_i : p_i = p_1$ versus the alternative hypothesis $H_i^A : p_i > p_1$. We put

$$\mathscr{H}_4 = \{H_i \mid i \in \mathscr{I}_{2,k}\}. \tag{7.4}$$

Under the condition (A3), for ℓ such that $2 \leq \ell \leq k$, we define T_ℓ and $\hat{\mu}_\ell$ by

$$T_\ell = \frac{\hat{\mu}_\ell - \hat{v}_1}{\sqrt{\frac{1}{n_2} + \frac{1}{n_1}}} \text{ and } \hat{\mu}_\ell = \max_{2 \leq s \leq \ell} \frac{\sum_{i=s}^{\ell} \hat{v}_i}{\ell - s + 1},$$

respectively, where $\hat{v}_i := 2 \arcsin\left(\sqrt{\hat{p}_i}\right)$.

Assume that $W_1, Z_2, \ldots, Z_k$ are independent and that $W_1 \sim N(0, \lambda_2/\lambda_1)$ and $Z_i \sim N(0, 1)$. We set

$$D_2(t|\ell, \lambda_2/\lambda_1) = P\left(\frac{\hat{\mu}_\ell^\Diamond - W_1}{\sqrt{1 + \lambda_2/\lambda_1}} \le t\right),\tag{7.5}$$

where $\hat{\mu}_\ell^\Diamond = \max_{2 \le s \le \ell}\left\{\left(\sum_{i=s}^\ell Z_i\right)/(\ell - s + 1)\right\}$. Then under H_0, $\lim_{n \to \infty} P_0$ $(T_\ell \le t) = D_2(t|\ell, \lambda_2/\lambda_1)$ holds. We denote the solution of $D_2(t) = 1 - \alpha$ by $d_2(\ell, \lambda_2/\lambda_1; \alpha)$, i.e., $D_2(d_2(\ell, \lambda_2/\lambda_1; \alpha)) = 1 - \alpha$. When the assumption (A2) of Sect. 6.3 is satisfied, for $\alpha = 0.05$, 0.025, 0.01, the values of $d_2(\ell, 1; \alpha)$ are stated in Tables 1 and 2 of Williams (1971). Shiraishi and Sugiura (2015) give the algorithm based on sinc method to calculate $d_2(\ell, 1; \alpha)$. The sinc method is described in Lund and Bowers (1992) and Stenger (1993). The algorithm is more efficient than that of Williams (1971).

[7.1] The Williams-Type Procedure

Whenever $d_2(\ell, \lambda_2/\lambda_1; \alpha) < T_\ell$ holds for any integer ℓ such that $i \le \ell \le k$, we reject the null hypothesis H_i.

Furthermore, we put $\mathscr{I}_\ell := \{i \mid 1 \le i \le \ell\}$ $(\ell = 2, \ldots, k)$. For $\ell = 2, \ldots, k$, we define $(\hat{v}_1^*(\mathscr{I}_\ell), \ldots, \hat{v}_\ell^*(\mathscr{I}_\ell))$ by $(u_1, \ldots, u_\ell)$ which minimize $\sum_{i=1}^\ell \lambda_{ni}(u_i - \hat{v}_i)^2$ under simple order restrictions $u_1 \le u_2 \le \ldots \le u_\ell$, i.e.,

$$\sum_{i=1}^\ell \lambda_{ni}\left(\hat{v}_i^*(\mathscr{I}_\ell) - \hat{v}_i\right)^2 = \min_{u_1 \le \ldots \le u_\ell} \sum_{i=1}^\ell \lambda_{ni}\left(u_i - \hat{v}_i\right)^2,$$

where $\lambda_{ni} := n_i/n$ and $n := n_1 + \ldots + n_k$. Let us put

$$\bar{\chi}_\ell^2(\mathscr{I}_\ell) := \sum_{i=1}^\ell n_i\left(\hat{v}_i^*(\mathscr{I}_\ell) - \sum_{i=1}^\ell \left(\frac{n_i}{n(\mathscr{I}_\ell)}\right)\hat{v}_i\right)^2 \quad (\ell = 2, \ldots, k),\tag{7.6}$$

where $n(\mathscr{I}_\ell) := \sum_{i=1}^\ell n_i$. We define $\tilde{v}_1^*(\mathscr{I}_\ell), \ldots, \tilde{v}_\ell^*(\mathscr{I}_\ell)$ by

$$\sum_{i=1}^\ell \lambda_i\left(\tilde{v}_i^*(\mathscr{I}_\ell) - Y_i\right)^2 = \min_{u_1 \le \ldots \le u_\ell} \sum_{i=1}^\ell \lambda_i(u_i - Y_i)^2,$$

where Y_i is defined in (6.3). $P(L, \ell; \lambda(\mathscr{I}_\ell))$ becomes the probability that $\tilde{v}_1^*(\mathscr{I}_\ell), \ldots,$ $\tilde{v}_\ell^*(\mathscr{I}_\ell)$ takes exactly L distinct values, where $\lambda(\mathscr{I}_\ell) = (\lambda_1, \ldots, \lambda_\ell)$. From the discussion similar to (6.3), we get, under (A1),

$$\lim_{n \to \infty} P_0(\bar{\chi}_\ell^2(\mathscr{I}_\ell) \ge t) = \sum_{L=2}^\ell P(L, \ell; \lambda(\mathscr{I}_\ell))P\left(\chi_{L-1}^2 \ge t\right) \quad (t > 0).\tag{7.7}$$

For a given α such that $0 < \alpha < 1$, we put

$\bar{c}^2 (\ell, \lambda(\mathcal{I}_\ell); \alpha) :=$ a solution of t satisfying the equation

$$\sum_{L=2}^{\ell} P(L, \ell; \lambda(\mathcal{I}_\ell)) P\left(\chi^2_{L-1} \geq t\right) = \alpha.$$

Then, we propose a stepwise procedure.

[7.2] Stepwise $\bar{\chi}^2$ Procedure
Whenever $\bar{c}^2 (\ell, \lambda(\mathcal{I}_\ell); \alpha) < \bar{\chi}^2_\ell(\mathcal{I}_\ell)$ holds for any integer ℓ such that $i \leq \ell \leq k$, we reject the null hypothesis H_i.

Theorem 7.1 *Under (A1), the level for test procedure [7.2] is asymptotically α as a multiple comparison test.*

Proof We put

$$\Theta_0 := \{\boldsymbol{p}| \text{ there exists integer } i \text{ such that } p_1 = p_i \text{ and } 2 \leq i \leq k\},$$

where $\boldsymbol{p} = (p_1, \cdots, p_k)$. We take any $\boldsymbol{p} \in \Theta_0$ and we put $i_0 := \max\{i| \ p_i = p_1\}$. We define D_ℓ by

$$D_\ell = \left\{\bar{c}^2 (\ell, \lambda(\mathcal{I}_\ell); \alpha) < \bar{\chi}^2_\ell(\mathcal{I}_\ell)\right\}.$$

For integer i satisfying $2 \leq i \leq i_0$, the event that the procedure [7.2] rejects the null hypothesis H_i is given by $\bigcap_{\ell=i}^{k} D_\ell$. The family-wise error rate of the procedure [7.2] is equal to

$$P_{\boldsymbol{p}} \left(\bigcup_{i=2}^{i_0} \left\{\bigcap_{\ell=i}^{k} D_\ell\right\}\right) \leq P_{\boldsymbol{p}} \left(D_{i_0}\right) = P_0 \left(D_{i_0}\right) \leq \alpha.$$

Hence, the assertion of the theorem is proved.   □

When the assumption (A2) of same sample sizes is satisfied, $\bar{c}^2 (\ell, \lambda(I); \alpha)$ does not depend on $\lambda(I)$ for $(\ell, I) = (\ell_1, I_1), \ldots, (\ell_J, I_J)$. Hence, under (A2), we rewrite $\bar{c}^2 (\ell, \lambda(I); \alpha)$ as $\bar{c}^2 (\ell, \alpha)$ shortly. Table 7.1 shows the critical values for $\alpha = 0.05$ or 0.01.

7.3 Successive Comparisons Between Ordered Proportions

We assume that the ordered restriction (7.1) is satisfied. In one comparison, we test the null hypothesis $H_{(i,i+1)} : \ p_i = p_{i+1}$ versus the alternative hypothesis $H^A_{(i,i+1)} : p_i < p_{i+1}$. We define $\widehat{T}_i(\boldsymbol{p})$ and $\widehat{T}_i$ by

Table 7.1 Critical values $\bar{c}^2(\ell, \alpha)$ for the proposed stepwise procedure for $\lambda_1 = \ldots = \lambda_k$

(a) $\alpha = 0.05$

ℓ	2	3	4	5	6	7	8	9	10
$\bar{c}^2(\ell, \alpha)$	2.706	3.820	4.528	5.049	5.460	5.800	6.088	6.339	6.560

(b) $\alpha = 0.01$

ℓ	2	3	4	5	6	7	8	9	10
$\bar{c}^2(\ell, \alpha)$	5.412	6.823	7.709	8.356	8.865	9.284	9.638	9.945	10.216

$$\widehat{T}_i(\boldsymbol{p}) := \frac{2\arcsin\left(\sqrt{\widehat{p}_{i+1}}\right) - 2\arcsin\left(\sqrt{\widehat{p}_i}\right) - 2\arcsin\left(\sqrt{p_{i+1}}\right) + 2\arcsin\left(\sqrt{p_i}\right)}{\sqrt{\frac{1}{n_{i+1}} + \frac{1}{n_i}}},$$

$$\widehat{T}_i := \widehat{T}_i(0) = \frac{2\arcsin\left(\sqrt{\widehat{p}_{i+1}}\right) - 2\arcsin\left(\sqrt{\widehat{p}_i}\right)}{\sqrt{\frac{1}{n_{i+1}} + \frac{1}{n_i}}},$$

respectively. From Lee and Spurrier (1995), by using $\max_{1 \le i \le k-1} \widehat{T}_i(\boldsymbol{p})$, we may state single-step multiple comparison procedures. Let us put

$$D_3(t) := P\left(\max_{1 \le i \le k-1} \frac{Y_{i+1} - Y_i}{\sqrt{\frac{1}{\lambda_{i+1}} + \frac{1}{\lambda_i}}} \le t\right), \tag{7.8}$$

where $Y_i \sim N(0, 1/\lambda_i)$ $(i = 1, \ldots, k)$ and $Y_1, \ldots, Y_k$ are independent. Then, from (6.3), we find

$$\lim_{n \to \infty} P\left(\max_{1 \le i \le k-1} \widehat{T}_i(\boldsymbol{p}) \le t\right) = \lim_{n \to \infty} P_0\left(\max_{1 \le i \le k-1} \widehat{T}_i \le t\right) = D_3(t).$$

From Liu et al. (2000), we can get the value of $D_2(t)$ by using the recurrence relation

$$h_3(t, y) = \int_{y-t\sqrt{1/\lambda_3 + 1/\lambda_2}}^{\infty} \left\{1 - \Phi\left(\sqrt{\lambda_1} \cdot y_2 - t\sqrt{\frac{\lambda_1}{\lambda_2} + 1}\right)\right\} \cdot \sqrt{\lambda_2}\varphi(\sqrt{\lambda_2} \cdot y_2)dy_2,$$

$$h_{r+1}(t, y) = \int_{y-t\sqrt{1/\lambda_{r+1} + 1/\lambda_r}}^{\infty} h_r(t, y_r) \cdot \sqrt{\lambda_r}\varphi(\sqrt{\lambda_r} \cdot y_r)dy_r \ (3 \le r \le k-1),$$

$$D_3(t) = \int_{-\infty}^{\infty} h_k(t, y)\sqrt{\lambda_k}\varphi(\sqrt{\lambda_k} \cdot y)dy, \tag{7.9}$$

where $\varphi(y)$ denotes a standard normal density function.

We denote the solution of $D_3(t) = 1 - \alpha$ by $d_3(k, \lambda_1, \ldots, \lambda_k; \alpha)$, i.e., $D_3(d_3(k, \lambda_1, \ldots, \lambda_k; \alpha)) = 1 - \alpha$.

By using $d_3(k, \lambda_1, \ldots, \lambda_k; \alpha)$, we may derive Lee-Spurrier-type single-step multiple comparison procedures [7.3] and [7.4].

[7.3] Asymptotic Simultaneous Intervals

The asymptotic $100(1 - \alpha)\%$ simultaneous lower confidence intervals for $\{\arcsin\left(\sqrt{p_{i+1}}\right) - \arcsin\left(\sqrt{p_i}\right) \mid i \in \mathscr{I}_{1,k-1}\}$ are given by

$$
\arcsin\left(\sqrt{\hat{p}_{i+1}}\right) - \arcsin\left(\sqrt{\hat{p}_i}\right) - d_3(k, \lambda_1, \ldots, \lambda_k; \alpha)\sqrt{\frac{1}{4n_{i+1}} + \frac{1}{4n_i}}
$$
$$
< \arcsin\left(\sqrt{p_{i+1}}\right) - \arcsin\left(\sqrt{p_i}\right) < \frac{\pi}{2} \quad (i \in \mathscr{I}_{1,k-1}).
$$

[7.4] Lee-Spurrier-Type Single-Step Simultaneous Test

The Lee-Spurrier-type test of level α for {the null hypothesis $H_{(i,i+1)}$ versus the alternative $H_{(i,i+1)}^A \mid i \in \mathscr{I}_{1,k-1}\}$ consists in rejecting $H_{(i,i+1)}$ for $i \in \mathscr{I}_{1,k-1}$ such that $\widehat{T}_i > d_3(k, \lambda_1, \ldots, \lambda_k; \alpha)$.

When $n_1 = \ldots = n_k$ is satisfied, $\lambda_1 = \ldots = \lambda_k = 1/k$ holds. Tables for the values of $d_3(k, 1/k, \ldots, 1/k; \alpha)$ appeared in Lee and Spurrier (1995).

Next, we discuss closed testing procedures. Let us put $\mathscr{V}_k := \{(i, i + 1) \mid i \in \mathscr{I}_{1,k-1}\}$ and

$$
\mathscr{H}_5 := \{H_{(i,i+1)} \mid i \in \mathscr{I}_{1,k-1}\}. \tag{7.10}
$$

Then, the closure of $\mathscr{H}_5$ is given by

$$
\overline{\mathscr{H}_5} = \left\{ \bigwedge_{v \in V} H_v \mid \emptyset \subsetneq V \subset \mathscr{V}_k \right\},
$$

where $\bigwedge$ denotes the conjunction symbol (Refer to Enderton (2001)). Then, we get

$$
\bigwedge_{v \in V} H_v : \text{for any } (i, i + 1) \in V, \ p_i = p_{i+1} \text{ holds.} \tag{7.11}
$$

Let $I_1, \ldots, I_J$ be disjoint sets satisfying the following property (P_3).

(P_3) There exist integers $\ell_1, \ldots, \ell_J \geq 2$ and integers $0 \leq s_1 < \ldots < s_J < k$ such that

$$
I_j = \{s_j + 1, s_j + 2, \ldots, s_j + \ell_j\} \ (j = 1, \ldots, J),
$$

$$
s_j + \ell_j \leq s_{j+1} \ (j = 1, \ldots, J - 1) \text{ and } s_J \leq k.
$$

We define the null hypothesis $H^O(I_1, \ldots, I_J)$ by

$$
H^O(I_1, \ldots, I_J) : \text{for any } j \text{ such that } 1 \leq j \leq J \text{ and for any } i, i' \in I_j,
$$
$$
p_i = p_{i'} \text{ holds.} \tag{7.12}
$$

The elements of I_j are consecutive integers and $\#(I_j) \geq 2$. From (7.11) and (7.12), for any nonempty $V \subset \mathcal{V}_k$, there exist an integer J and some subsets $I_1, \ldots, I_J \subset \{1, \ldots, k\}$ satisfying (P_3) such that

$$\bigwedge_{v \in V} H_v = H^O(I_1, \ldots, I_J). \tag{7.13}$$

Furthermore, $H^O(I_1, \ldots, I_J)$ is expressed as

$$H^O(I_1, \ldots, I_J) : \; p_{s_j+1} = p_{s_j+2} = \ldots = p_{s_j+\ell_j} \; (j = 1, \ldots, J). \tag{7.14}$$

For $H^O(I_1, \ldots, I_J)$ of (7.13), we set

$$M = M(I_1, \ldots, I_J) = \sum_{j=1}^{J} \ell_j, \; \ell_j = \#(I_j). \tag{7.15}$$

For $j = 1, \ldots, J$, we put

$$D_3(t|I_j) := P\left(\max_{s_j+1 \leq i \leq s_j+\ell_j-1} \frac{Y_{i+1} - Y_i}{\sqrt{\frac{1}{\lambda_{i+1}} + \frac{1}{\lambda_i}}} \leq t \right), \tag{7.16}$$

where Y_i's are defined in (7.8). We denote the solution of $D_3(t|I_j) = 1 - \alpha$ by $d_3(\ell_j, I_j; \alpha)$, i.e., $D_3(d_3(\ell_j, I_j; \alpha)|I_j) = 1 - \alpha$.

Then, we propose a stepwise procedure.

[7.5] Stepwise Procedure
The assumption (A2) of same sample sizes is assumed. For $\ell = \ell_1, \ldots, \ell_J$, we define $\alpha(M, \ell)$ by

$$\alpha(M, \ell) = 1 - (1 - \alpha)^{\ell/M}.$$

We put

$$\widehat{T}(I_j) := \max_{s_j+1 \leq i \leq s_j+\ell_j-1} \widehat{T}_i \; (j = 1, \ldots, J).$$

(a) $J \geq 2$
   Whenever $d_3\left(\ell_j, I_j; \alpha(M, \ell_j)\right) < \widehat{T}(I_j)$ holds for an integer j such that $1 \leq j \leq J$, we reject the hypothesis $\bigwedge_{v \in V} H_v$.

(b) $J = 1 \; (M = \ell_1)$
   Whenever $d_3\left(\ell_1, I_1; \alpha\right) < \widehat{T}(I_1)$, we reject the hypothesis $\bigwedge_{v \in V} H_v$.

By using the methods of (a) and (b), when $\bigwedge_{\nu \in V} H_\nu$ is rejected for any V such that $(i, i+1) \in V \subset \mathcal{V}_k$, the null hypothesis $H_{(i,i+1)}$ is rejected as a multiple comparison test. Then, this procedure also becomes a closed test.

Theorem 7.2 *Under (A1), the level for test procedure [7.5] is asymptotically α as a multiple comparison test.*

Proof It is trivial to verify that the level of the test procedure of (b) is α. We show that the level of the test procedure of (a) is α. Furthermore, we suppose without any loss of generality that H_0 is true. Since $\widehat{T}(I_1), \ldots, \widehat{T}(I_J)$ are independent, we get

$$\lim_{n \to \infty} P_0 \left(\widehat{T}(I_j) < d_3 \left(\ell_j, I_j; \alpha(M, \ell_j) \right), \; j = 1, \ldots, J \right)$$

$$= \prod_{j=1}^{J} \left\{ \lim_{n \to \infty} P_0 \left(\widehat{T}(I_j) < d_3 \left(\ell_j, I_j; \alpha(M, \ell_j) \right) \right) \right\}. \tag{7.17}$$

By using

$$\lim_{n \to \infty} P_0 \left(\widehat{T}(I_j) < t \right) = D_3(t | I_j),$$

we have

$$(7.17) = \prod_{j=1}^{J} D_3 \left(d_3 \left(\ell_j, I_j; \alpha(M, \ell_j) \right) | I_j \right)$$

$$= \prod_{j=1}^{J} \left(1 - \alpha(M, \ell_j) \right)$$

$$= \prod_{j=1}^{J} \left\{ (1 - \alpha)^{\ell_j / M} \right\}$$

$$= 1 - \alpha. \tag{7.18}$$

From (7.18), we have

$$\lim_{n \to \infty} P_0 \left(\text{There exists } j \text{ such that } \widehat{T}(I_j) \geq d_3 \left(\ell_j, I_j; \alpha(M, \ell_j) \right) \right)$$

$$= 1 - \lim_{n \to \infty} P_0 \left(\widehat{T}(I_j) < d_3 \left(\ell_j, I_j; \alpha(M, \ell_j) \right), \; j = 1, \ldots, J \right).$$

$$= \alpha$$

Therefore, the level of the test procedure of (a) for the null hypothesis $\bigwedge_{\nu \in V} H_\nu$ is asymptotically α. Hence, the assertion of the theorem is proved. $\qquad \square$

Table 7.2 The values of $d_3(k; \alpha)$ for $\alpha = 0.05, 0.01$ and $k = 3(1)10$

$100\alpha\% \setminus k$	3	4	5	6	7	8	9	10
5%	1.960	2.126	2.238	2.322	2.389	2.444	2.492	2.533
1%	2.576	2.713	2.806	2.877	2.934	2.982	3.022	3.058

Table 7.3 The values of $d_3(\ell; \alpha(M, \ell))$ for $\alpha = 0.05$ and $M = 2(1)10$

$M \setminus \ell$	2	3	4	5	6	7	8	9	10
10	2.319	2.426	2.468	2.491	2.506	2.516	2.523	◊	2.533
9	2.279	2.388	2.431	2.454	2.469	2.479	◊	2.492	
8	2.234	2.345	2.388	2.412	2.427	◊	2.444		
7	2.182	2.295	2.339	2.363	◊	2.389			
6	2.121	2.236	2.282	◊	2.322				
5	2.047	2.166	◊	2.238					
4	1.955	◊	2.126						
3	◊	1.960							
2	1.645								

The places of ◊ are not used in the procedure [7.5]. As an example, $d_3(3; \alpha(7, 3)) = 2.295$

From (7.8), since $d_3(k, \lambda_1, \ldots, \lambda_k; \alpha)$ depends on k and α for

$$\lambda_1 = \ldots = \lambda_k = 1/k, \tag{7.19}$$

$d_3(k, 1/k, \ldots, 1/k; \alpha)$ is abbreviated as $d_3(k; \alpha)$. When sample sizes are equal, that is,

$$n_1 = \ldots = n_k, \tag{7.20}$$

(7.19) is satisfied. The values of $d_3(k; \alpha)$ for $\alpha = 0.05, 0.01$ and $k = 3(1)10$ are provided in Table 7.2. Similarly, from (7.16), since $d_3(\ell_j, I_j; \alpha(M, \ell_j))$ depends on ℓ_j and α for (7.19), $d_3(\ell_j, I_j; \alpha(M, \ell_j))$ is abbreviated as $d_3(\ell_j; \alpha(M, \ell_j))$ under (7.19). For $\alpha = 0.05, 0.01$, we give the values of $d_3(\ell; \alpha(M, \ell))$ in Tables 7.3 and 7.4, respectively. We limited attention to $2 \le M \le 10$. $\ell = M - 1$ is not used in the procedure [7.5]. When $\ell = M = k$ is satisfied, $d_3(\ell; \alpha(M, \ell)) = d_3(k; \alpha)$ holds.

For $\alpha = 0.05, 0.01$ and $4 \le k \le 10$, from Tables 7.2, 7.3, and 7.4, we find

$$d_3(\ell; \alpha(M, \ell)) < d_3(k; \alpha(k, k)) = d_3(k; \alpha) \tag{7.21}$$

for ℓ such that $2 \le \ell < M \le k$. By numerical calculation, we verify that (7.21) holds for $\alpha = 0.05, 0.01$ and $3 \le k \le 10$. From the construction of the closed testing procedure [7.5] and the relation of (7.21), we get the following (i) and (ii). (i) The procedure [7.5] of level α rejects $H_{(i,i+1)}$ that is rejected by the single-step simultaneous test [7.4] of level α. (ii) The single-step simultaneous test [7.4] of level α does

Table 7.4 The values of d_3 $(\ell; \alpha(M, \ell))$ for $\alpha = 0.01$ and $M = 2(1)10$

$M \setminus \ell$	2	3	4	5	6	7	8	9	10
10	2.877	2.967	3.003	3.022	3.035	3.043	3.049	◊	3.058
9	2.844	2.934	2.971	2.990	3.003	3.011	◊	3.022	
8	2.806	2.897	2.934	2.954	2.967	◊	2.982		
7	2.763	2.855	2.893	2.913	◊	2.934			
6	2.712	2.806	2.844	◊	2.877				
5	2.651	2.747	◊	2.806					
4	2.575	◊	2.713						
3	◊	2.576							
2	2.326								

not always reject $H_{(i,i'+1)}$ that is rejected by the procedure [7.5] of level α. Hence, for $\alpha = 0.05,\ 0.01$ and $3 \le k \le 10$, the closed testing procedure [7.5] is more powerful than the single-step simultaneous test [7.4].

We get Theorem 7.3 as in the proof of Theorem 3.3.

Theorem 7.3 *Let* $A'_{(i,i+1)}$ *be the event that* $H_{(i,i+1)}$ *is rejected by the procedure [7.5] as a multiple comparison of level* α $(i \in \mathscr{I}_{1,k-1})$. *Suppose that*

$$d_3 \left(\ell; \alpha(M, \ell) \right) < d_3(k; \alpha) \tag{7.22}$$

is satisfied for any M *such that* $4 \le M \le k$ *and any integer* ℓ *such that* $2 \le \ell \le M - 2$, *where* M *is defined by (7.15). Then the following relations hold.*

$$P \left(\bigcup_{i=1}^{k-1} A'_{(i,i+1)} \right) = P \left(\max_{1 \le i \le k-1} \widehat{T}_i > d_3(k; \alpha) \right)$$

$$P \left(A'_{(i,i+1)} \right) \ge P \left(\widehat{T}_i > d_3(k; \alpha) \right) \quad \left(i \in \mathscr{I}_{1,k-1} \right).$$

$\square$

References

Agresti A, Coull BA (1996) Order-restricted tests for stratified comparisons of binomial proportions. Biometrics 52:1103–1111

Chernoff H (1954) On the distribution of the likelihood ratio. Ann Math Statist 25:573–578

Lee RE, Spurrier JD (1995) Successive comparisons between ordered treatments. J Statist Plann Infer 43:323–330

Liu W, Miwa T, Hayter AJ (2000) Simultaneous confidence interval estimation for successive comparisons of ordered treatment effects. J Statist Plann Infer 88:75–86

Lund J, Bowers KL (1992) Sinc methods for quadrature and differential equations. Siam

Shiraishi T, Sugiura H (2015) The upper $100\alpha^*$th percentiles of the distributions used in multiple comparison procedures under a simple order restriction. J Japan Statist Soc 44:271–314 (in Japanese)

Stenger F (1993) Numerical methods based on Sinc and analytic function. Springer

Williams DA (1971) A test for differences between treatment means when several dose levels are compared with a zero dose control. Biometrics 27:103–117

Williams DA (1972) The comparison of several dose levels are compared with a zero dose control. Biometrics 28:519–531

Chapter 8
Hybrid Serial Gatekeeping Procedures for All-Pairwise Comparisons

Abstract In q multi-sample models, we consider multiple comparison tests for all-pairwise differences of proportions. Let $\mathcal{H}_1^{(r)}$ be the family of null hypothesis among $k^{(r)}$ proportions for $r = 1, \ldots, q$. The family $\mathcal{H}_1^{(1)} \succ \ldots \succ \mathcal{H}_1^{(q)}$ has the order of priority. This chapter describes procedures for performing multiple comparison tests at level α based on serial gatekeeping methods. In the r-th stage, a test procedure under unrestricted proportions or a test procedure under order restricted proportions is used. The proposed hybrid procedures are the methods assuming the Bernoulli distribution. The power of the proposed tests is much superior to the serial gatekeeping methods based on Bonferroni tests which are proposed by Mauer (1995).

8.1 Introduction

We consider k-sample models with Bernoulli responses. $(X_{i1}, \ldots, X_{in_i})$ is a random sample of size n_i from the i-th Bernoulli population with success probability p_i $(i = 1, \ldots, k)$. It is convenient to assign the number 1 to a success and the number 0 to a failure.

$$P(X_{ij} = 1) = p_i \quad \text{and} \quad P(X_{ij} = 0) = 1 - p_i$$

hold. X_{ij}'s are assumed to be independent. Chapter 3 discussed Tukey-Kramer-type single-step procedures [3.1] as multiple comparison tests of level α for all-pairwise comparisons of $\{$the null hypothesis $H_{(i,i')} : p_i = p_{i'}$ versus the alternative $H_{(i,i')}^A : p_i \neq p_{i'} \mid (i, i') \in \mathcal{U}_k\}$, where $\mathcal{U}_k := \{(i, i') \mid 1 \leq i < i' \leq k\}$. As multi-step procedures, Chap. 3 discussed closed testing procedures.

When the simple order restrictions

$$p_1 \leq p_2 \leq \ldots \leq p_k \tag{8.1}$$

© The Author(s), under exclusive license to Springer Nature Singapore Pte Ltd. 2022
T. Shiraishi, *Multiple Comparisons for Bernoulli Data*,
JSS Research Series in Statistics,
https://doi.org/10.1007/978-981-19-2708-9_8

are satisfied, Chap. 6 stated Hayter-type single-step simultaneous tests for {the null hypothesis $H_{(i,i')}$ versus the alternative $H_{(i,i')}^{OA} : p_i < p_{i'} | (i, i') \in \mathcal{U}_k$} under the equal sample sizes $n_1 = \ldots = n_k$. Furthermore, Chap. 6 proposed closed testing procedures and showed that the proposed multi-step procedures are more powerful than the single-step procedures.

Gatekeeping procedures became to be used in recent years as a convenient way to handle relationships between multiple hierarchical objectives. To solve questions concerning different objectives, null hypotheses are divided into q ordered families, $\mathcal{F}^{(1)} \succ \ldots \succ \mathcal{F}^{(q)}$. Westfall and Krishen (2001) proposed the serial gatekeeping procedures in which the hypotheses in $\mathcal{F}^{(r+1)}$ are tested if and only if all hypotheses in $\mathcal{F}^{(r)}$ are rejected ($1 \leq r \leq q - 1$). The individual test procedures are based on Bonferroni tests.

In this chapter, we consider q multi-sample models. In the r-th multi-sample models, $\left(X_{i1}^{(r)}, \ldots, X_{in_i^{(r)}}^{(r)} \right)$ is a random sample of size $n_i^{(r)}$ from the i-th Bernoulli population with success probability $p_i^{(r)}$ ($i = 1, \ldots, k^{(r)}$). It is convenient to assign the number 1 to a success and the number 0 to a failure.

$$P(X_{ij}^{(r)} = 1) = p_i^{(r)} \text{ and } P(X_{ij}^{(r)} = 0) = 1 - p_i^{(r)}$$

hold. $X_{i1}^{(r)}, \ldots, X_{in_i^{(r)}}^{(r)}$ are assumed to be independent. We need not assume that $X^{(1)}, \ldots, X^{(q)}$ are independent, where $X^{(r)} := \left(X_{11}^{(r)}, \ldots, X_{k^{(r)} n_{k^{(r)}}^{(r)}}^{(r)} \right)$. Let

$$\mathcal{H}_1^{(r)} := \left\{ H_{ii'}^{(r)} : p_i^{(r)} = p_{i'}^{(r)} \middle| (i, i') \in \mathcal{U}_{k^{(r)}} \right\} \tag{8.2}$$

be the family of null hypothesis among $k^{(r)}$ proportions for $r = 1, \ldots, q$, where

$$\mathcal{U}_{k^{(r)}} := \{(i, i') \mid 1 \leq i < i' \leq k^{(r)}\}. \tag{8.3}$$

The family $\mathcal{H}_1^{(1)}, \ldots, \mathcal{H}_1^{(q)}$ has the order of priority.

$$\mathcal{H}_1^{(1)} \succ \ldots \succ \mathcal{H}_1^{(q)}. \tag{8.4}$$

This paper describes procedures for performing multiple comparison tests at level α based on serial gatekeeping methods. In the r-th stage, a test procedure under unrestricted proportions or a test procedure under order restricted proportions is used. The methods of procedures [3.1], [3.3], [3.5], [6.2], [6.3], and [6.4] stated in Chaps. 3 and 6 are used in the hybrid gatekeeping procedures. The power of the proposed tests is much superior to the serial gatekeeping methods based on Bonferroni tests which are usually used.

8.2 Multiple Comparisons Under Unrestricted Proportions in the r-th Multi-sample Model

For specified i, i' such that $1 \leq i < i' \leq k^{(r)}$, if we are interested in testing the null hypothesis $H^{(r)}_{(i,i')} : p_i^{(r)} = p_{i'}^{(r)}$ versus the alternative $H^{(r)A}_{(i,i')} : p_i^{(r)} \neq p_{i'}^{(r)}$, we can use the two-sided two-sample tests. In this section, we consider test procedures for all-pairwise comparisons of

$$\{\text{the null hypothesis } H^{(r)}_{(i,i')} \text{ versus the alternative } H^{(r)A}_{(i,i')} \,|\, (i, i') \in \mathcal{U}_{k^{(r)}}\}, \qquad (8.5)$$

where $\mathcal{U}_{k^{(r)}}$ is defined by (8.3). We add the assumption of

$$(A4) \qquad \lim_{n^{(r)} \to \infty} \frac{n_i^{(r)}}{n^{(r)}} = \lambda_i^{(r)} > 0, \quad (1 \leq i \leq k^{(r)}),$$

where $n^{(r)} := \sum_{i=1}^{k} n_i^{(r)}$. We introduce two distribution functions of $A(t|k^{(r)})$ and $A^*(t|k^{(r)}, \lambda^{(r)})$.

$$A(t|k^{(r)}) := k^{(r)} \int_{-\infty}^{\infty} \{\Phi(x) - \Phi(x - \sqrt{2} \cdot t)\}^{k^{(r)}-1} d\Phi(x), \qquad (8.6)$$

$$A^*(t|k^{(r)}, \lambda^{(r)}) := \sum_{j=1}^{k^{(r)}} \int_{-\infty}^{\infty} \prod_{\substack{i=1 \\ i \neq j}}^{k^{(r)}} \left\{ \Phi\left(\sqrt{\frac{\lambda_i^{(r)}}{\lambda_j^{(r)}}} \cdot x \right) \right.$$
$$\left. - \Phi\left(\sqrt{\frac{\lambda_i^{(r)}}{\lambda_j^{(r)}}} \cdot x - \sqrt{\frac{\lambda_i^{(r)} + \lambda_j^{(r)}}{\lambda_j^{(r)}}} \cdot t \right) \right\} d\Phi(x),$$

where

$$\lambda^{(r)} := (\lambda_1^{(r)}, \ldots, \lambda_{k^{(r)}}^{(r)}) \quad (r = 1, \ldots, q). \qquad (8.7)$$

We put

$$T_{i'i}^{(r)} := \frac{2 \left\{ \arcsin\left(\sqrt{\hat{p}_{i'}^{(r)}} \right) - \arcsin\left(\sqrt{\hat{p}_i^{(r)}} \right) \right\}}{\sqrt{\frac{1}{n_i^{(r)}} + \frac{1}{n_{i'}^{(r)}}}}, \qquad ((i, i') \in \mathcal{U}_{k^{(r)}}), \qquad (8.8)$$

where

$$\hat{p}_i^{(r)} := \frac{X_{i\cdot}^{(r)}}{n_i^{(r)}} \quad \text{or} \quad \frac{X_{i\cdot}^{(r)} + 0.5}{n_i^{(r)} + 1} \qquad (8.9)$$

and $X_{i\cdot}^{(r)} := \sum_{j=1}^{n_i^{(r)}} X_{ij}^{(r)}$. Then we get, for $t > 0$,

$$A(t|k^{(r)}) \leq \lim_{n^{(r)} \to \infty} P_{(r)0}\left(\max_{(i,i') \in \mathcal{U}_{k^{(r)}}} |T_{i'i}^{(r)}| \leq t\right) \leq A^*(t|k^{(r)}, \boldsymbol{\lambda}^{(r)}) \qquad (8.10)$$

holds, where $P_{(r)0}(\cdot)$ stands for probability measure under the following null hypothesis $H_0^{(r)}$.

$$H_0^{(r)} : \ p_1^{(r)} = \ldots = p_{k^{(r)}}^{(r)}. \qquad (8.11)$$

When $n_1^{(r)} = \ldots = n_{k^{(r)}}^{(r)}$ is satisfied, both of the inequalities of (8.10) become an equality.

The left-hand side of the inequality (8.10) is derived from the main theorem of Hayter (1984). The right-hand side of the inequality (8.10) is given by Shiraishi (2006). For a given α such that $0 < \alpha < 1$, we put

$$a(k^{(r)}; \alpha) := \text{a solution of } t \text{ satisfying the equation } A(t|k^{(r)}) = 1 - \alpha. \qquad (8.12)$$

[8.1] Single-Step Tests

The Tukey-Kramer-type simultaneous test of level α for the null hypotheses $\{H_{(i,i')}^{(r)}|$ $(i, i') \in \mathcal{U}_{k^{(r)}}\}$ consists in rejecting $H_{(i,i')}^{(r)}$ for $(i, i') \in \mathcal{U}_{k^{(r)}}$ such that $|T_{i'i}^{(r)}| > a(k^{(r)}; \alpha)$. From the left inequality of (8.10), we find that the Tukey-Kramer simultaneous test is conservative. Under the condition of $\max_{1 \leq i \leq k^{(r)}} n_i^{(r)} / \min_{1 \leq i \leq k^{(r)}} n_i^{(r)} \leq 2$, Shiraishi (2006) found that the values of $A^*(t|k^{(r)}, \boldsymbol{\lambda}^{(r)}) - A(t|k^{(r)})$ are nearly equal to 0 for various values of t from numerical integration. Therefore, the conservativeness of the Tukey-Kramer method is small.

The closure of $\mathscr{H}_1^{(r)}$ is given by

$$\overline{\mathscr{H}_1^{(r)}} = \left\{ \bigwedge_{v \in V} H_v^{(r)} \mid \emptyset \subsetneq V \subset \mathcal{U}_{k^{(r)}} \right\},$$

where $\bigwedge$ denotes the conjunction symbol (Refer to Enderton (2001)). Then, we get

$$\bigwedge_{v \in V} H_v^{(r)} : \text{for any } (i, i') \in V, \ p_i^{(r)} = p_{i'}^{(r)} \text{ holds.} \qquad (8.13)$$

For an integer $J^{(r)}$ and disjoint sets $I_1^{(r)}, \ldots, I_{J^{(r)}}^{(r)} \subset \{1, \ldots, k^{(r)}\}$, we define the null hypothesis $H^{(r)}(I_1^{(r)}, \ldots, I_{J^{(r)}}^{(r)})$ by

$$H^{(r)}(I_1^{(r)}, \ldots, I_{J^{(r)}}^{(r)}) : \text{for any integer } j \text{ such that } 1 \leq j \leq J^{(r)}$$
$$\text{and for any } i, i' \in I_j^{(r)}, \ p_i^{(r)} = p_{i'}^{(r)} \text{ holds.} \qquad (8.14)$$

From (8.13) and (8.14), for any nonempty $V \subset \mathcal{U}_{k^{(r)}}$, there exist an integer $J^{(r)}$ and disjoint sets $I_1^{(r)}, \ldots, I_{J^{(r)}}^{(r)}$ such that

$$\bigwedge_{v \in V} H_v^{(r)} = H^{(r)}(I_1^{(r)}, \ldots, I_{J^{(r)}}^{(r)}) \tag{8.15}$$

and $\#(I_j^{(r)}) \geq 2$ $(j = 1, \ldots, J^{(r)})$, where $\#(A)$ stands for the cardinal number of set A. For $H^{(r)}(I_1^{(r)}, \ldots, I_{J^{(r)}}^{(r)})$ of (8.15), we set

$$M^{(r)} := M^{(r)}(I_1^{(r)}, \ldots, I_{J^{(r)}}^{(r)}) = \sum_{j=1}^{J^{(r)}} \ell_j^{(r)}, \quad \ell_j^{(r)} := \#(I_j^{(r)}). \tag{8.16}$$

Let us put

$$T^{(r)}(I_j^{(r)}) := \max_{i < i', \, i,i' \in I_j^{(r)}} \left| T_{i'i}^{(r)} \right| \quad (j = 1, \ldots, J^{(r)}).$$

Then, we propose the stepwise procedure [8.2].

[8.2] Stepwise procedure
For $\ell^{(r)} = \ell_1^{(r)}, \ldots, \ell_{J^{(r)}}^{(r)}$, we define $\alpha(M^{(r)}, \ell^{(r)})$ by

$$\alpha(M^{(r)}, \ell^{(r)}) := 1 - (1 - \alpha)^{\ell^{(r)}/M^{(r)}}. \tag{8.17}$$

Corresponding to (8.6), we put

$$A(t|\ell^{(r)}) := \ell^{(r)} \int_{-\infty}^{\infty} \{\Phi(x) - \Phi(x - \sqrt{2} \cdot t)\}^{\ell^{(r)}-1} d\Phi(x).$$

By obeying the notation $a(k^{(r)}; \alpha)$, we get

$$A(a(\ell^{(r)}; \alpha(M^{(r)}, \ell^{(r)}))|\ell^{(r)}) = 1 - \alpha(M^{(r)}, \ell^{(r)}), \tag{8.18}$$

that is, $a(\ell^{(r)}; \alpha(M^{(r)}, \ell^{(r)}))$ is an upper $100\alpha(M^{(r)}, \ell^{(r)})\%$ point of the distribution $A(t|\ell^{(r)})$.

(a) $J^{(r)} \geq 2$
   Whenever $a\left(\ell_j^{(r)}; \alpha(M^{(r)}, \ell_j^{(r)})\right) < T^{(r)}(I_j^{(r)})$ holds for an integer j such that $1 \leq j \leq J^{(r)}$, we reject the hypothesis $\bigwedge_{v \in V} H_v^{(r)}$.
(b) $J^{(r)} = 1$ $(M^{(r)} = \ell_1^{(r)})$
   Whenever $a\left(M^{(r)}; \alpha\right) < T^{(r)}(I_1^{(r)})$ holds, we reject the hypothesis $\bigwedge_{v \in V} H_v^{(r)}$.

By using the methods of (a) and (b), when $\bigwedge_{v \in V} H_v^{(r)}$ is rejected for any V such that $(i, i') \in V \subset \mathcal{U}_{k^{(r)}}$, the null hypothesis $H_{(i,i')}^{(r)}$ is rejected as a multiple comparison test of level α.

[8.3] Stepwise Procedure Based on χ^2-Statistics

Let us put, for $j = 1, \ldots, J^{(r)}$,

$$
S^{(r)}(I_j^{(r)}) := 4 \sum_{i \in I_j^{(r)}} n_i^{(r)} \left\{ \arcsin\left(\sqrt{\hat{p}_i^{(r)}} \right) - \sum_{i' \in I_j^{(r)}} \left(\frac{n_{i'}^{(r)}}{n^{(r)}(I_j^{(r)})} \right) \arcsin\left(\sqrt{\hat{p}_{i'}^{(r)}} \right) \right\}^2,
$$

$$(8.19)$$

where $I_j^{(r)}$ is defined in (8.15) and $n^{(r)}(I_j^{(r)}) := \sum_{i \in I_j^{(r)}} n_i^{(r)}$. In the procedure [8.2], replace

$a\left(\ell_j^{(r)}; \alpha(M^{(r)}, \ell_j^{(r)}) \right) < T^{(r)}(I_j^{(r)})$ and $a\left(M^{(r)}; \alpha \right) < T^{(r)}(I_1^{(r)})$ with

$\chi^2_{\ell_j^{(r)}-1}\left(\alpha(M^{(r)}, \ell_j^{(r)}) \right) < S^{(r)}(I_j^{(r)})$ and $\chi^2_{M^{(r)}-1}(\alpha) < S(I_1^{(r)})$, respectively. Here, $\chi^2_{k-1}(\alpha)$ denotes the upper $100\alpha\%$ point of χ^2-distribution with $k - 1$ degrees of freedom. Then, this procedure also becomes a closed test of level α.

8.3 Comparisons Under Order Restricted Proportions in the r-th Multi-sample Model

When the simple order restrictions

$$
p_1^{(r)} \leq p_2^{(r)} \leq \cdots \leq p_{k^{(r)}}^{(r)} \tag{8.20}
$$

are satisfied, we consider the null hypothesis $H_0^{(r)}$ versus the alternative $H^{(r)A}$: $p_1^{(r)} \leq p_2^{(r)} \leq \cdots \leq p_{k^{(r)}}^{(r)}$ with at least one strict inequality, which is equivalent to $H_0^{(r)}$: $p_1^{(r)} = p_{k^{(r)}}^{(r)}$ versus $H^{(r)A}$: $p_1^{(r)} < p_{k^{(r)}}^{(r)}$, where $H_0^{(r)}$ is defined by (8.11). We put $\hat{v}_i^{(r)} := 2\arcsin\left(\sqrt{\hat{p}_i^{(r)}} \right)$ and $v_i^{(r)} = 2\arcsin\left(\sqrt{p_i^{(r)}} \right)$. Then using a central limit theorem and Slutsky's theorem, under (A4), we get

$$
\sqrt{n^{(r)}}\left(\hat{v}_i^{(r)} - v_i^{(r)} \right) \xrightarrow{\mathscr{L}} Y_i^{(r)} \sim N\left(0, \frac{1}{\lambda_i^{(r)}} \right). \tag{8.21}
$$

We define $\{\hat{v}_i^{(r)*} | i = 1, \ldots, k^{(r)}\}$ by $\{u_i | i = 1, \ldots, k^{(r)}\}$ which minimize $\sum_{i=1}^{k^{(r)}} \lambda_{ni}^{(r)} \left(u_i - \hat{v}_i^{(r)} \right)^2$ under simple order restrictions $u_1 \leq u_2 \leq \cdots \leq u_{k^{(r)}}$, i.e.,

$$
\sum_{i=1}^{k^{(r)}} \lambda_{ni}^{(r)} \left(\hat{v}_i^{(r)*} - \hat{v}_i^{(r)} \right)^2 = \min_{u_1 \leq \cdots \leq u_{k^{(r)}}} \sum_{i=1}^{k^{(r)}} \lambda_{ni}^{(r)} \left(u_i - \hat{v}_i^{(r)} \right)^2,
$$

where $\lambda_{ni}^{(r)} := n_i^{(r)}/n^{(r)}$ $(1 \leq i \leq k^{(r)})$. $\hat{v}_1^{(r)*}, \ldots, \hat{v}_{k^{(r)}}^{(r)*}$ are computed by using the pool-adjacent-violators algorithm stated in Robertson et al. (1988) and

$$\hat{v}_i^{(r)*} = \max_{1 \leq a \leq i} \min_{i \leq b \leq k^{(r)}} \frac{\sum_{j=a}^b \lambda_{nj}^{(r)} \hat{v}_j^{(r)}}{\sum_{j=a}^b \lambda_{nj}^{(r)}} = \max_{1 \leq a \leq i} \min_{i \leq b \leq k^{(r)}} \frac{\sum_{j=a}^b n_j^{(r)} \hat{v}_j^{(r)}}{\sum_{j=a}^b n_j^{(r)}} \qquad (8.22)$$

holds. We put

$$\bar{\chi}_{k^{(r)}}^2 := \sum_{i=1}^{k^{(r)}} n_i^{(r)} \left(\hat{v}_i^{(r)*} - \sum_{j=1}^{k^{(r)}} \lambda_{nj}^{(r)} \hat{v}_j^{(r)} \right)^2 .$$

We define $\tilde{v}_1^{(r)*}, \ldots, \tilde{v}_{k^{(r)}}^{(r)*}$ by

$$\sum_{i=1}^{k^{(r)}} \lambda_i^{(r)} \left(\tilde{v}_i^{(r)*} - Y_i^{(r)} \right)^2 = \min_{u_1 \leq \ldots \leq u_{k^{(r)}}} \sum_{i=1}^{k^{(r)}} \lambda_i^{(r)} \left(u_i - Y_i^{(r)} \right)^2 ,$$

where $Y_i^{(r)}$ is defined in (8.21). Let $P(L, k^{(r)}; \boldsymbol{\lambda}^{(r)})$ be the probability that $\tilde{v}_1^{(r)*}, \ldots,$ $\tilde{v}_{k^{(r)}}^{(r)*}$ takes exactly L distinct values, where $\boldsymbol{\lambda}^{(r)} := (\lambda_1^{(r)}, \ldots, \lambda_{k^{(r)}}^{(r)})$. Then, for positive constant c, $P(L, k^{(r)}; c\boldsymbol{\lambda}^{(r)}) = P(L, k^{(r)}; \boldsymbol{\lambda}^{(r)})$ holds. Furthermore, from Theorem 2.3.1 of Robertson et al. (1988), we get

$$\lim_{n^{(r)} \to \infty} P_{(r)0}(\bar{\chi}_{k^{(r)}}^2 \geq t) = \sum_{L=2}^{k^{(r)}} P(L, k^{(r)}; \boldsymbol{\lambda}^{(r)}) P\left(\chi_{L-1}^2 \geq t \right) \quad (t > 0), \qquad (8.23)$$

where $P_{(r)0}(\cdot)$ stands for probability measure under the null hypothesis $H_0^{(r)}$ of (8.11) and χ_{L-1}^2 is a chi-square variable with $L - 1$ degrees of freedom. The recurrence formula of computing $P(L, k^{(r)}; \boldsymbol{\lambda}^{(r)})$ is written in Robertson et al. (1988). The fundamental algorithm of $P(L, k^{(r)}; \boldsymbol{\lambda}^{(r)})$ based on sinc integral is stated in Sect. 7.4 of Shiraishi et al. (2019).

Since $P(L, k^{(r)}; \boldsymbol{\lambda}^{(r)})$ depends on L and $k^{(r)}$ for

$$\lambda_1^{(r)} = \ldots = \lambda_{k^{(r)}}^{(r)} = 1/k^{(r)}, \qquad (8.24)$$

we simply write $P(L, k^{(r)})$ instead of $P(L, k^{(r)}; \boldsymbol{\lambda}^{(r)})$. Barlow et al. (1972) offer the following recurrence formula.

$$P(1, k^{(r)}) = \frac{1}{k^{(r)}},$$

$$P(L, k^{(r)}) = \frac{1}{k^{(r)}} \left\{ (k^{(r)} - 1) P(L, k^{(r)} - 1) + P(L - 1, k^{(r)} - 1) \right\}, \qquad (2 \leq L \leq k^{(r)} - 1)$$

$$P(k^{(r)}, k^{(r)}) = \frac{1}{k^{(r)}!} .$$

For a given α such that $0 < \alpha < 1$, we give the following equation of t.

$$\sum_{L=2}^{k^{(r)}} P(L, k^{(r)}; \lambda^{(r)}) P\left(\chi^2_{L-1} \geq t\right) = \alpha.$$

We denote a solution of this equation by $\bar{c}^2(k^{(r)}, \lambda^{(r)}; \alpha)$. Hence, from (8.23), we can reject $H_0^{(r)}$ when the value of $\bar{\chi}^2_{k^{(r)}}$ is greater than $\bar{c}^2(k^{(r)}, \lambda^{(r)}; \alpha)$.

For specified i, i' such that $(i, i') \in \mathcal{U}_{k^{(r)}}$, if we are interested in testing of

the null hypothesis $H_{(i,i')}^{(r)} : p_i^{(r)} = p_{i'}^{(r)}$ versus the alternative $H_{(i,i')}^{(r)OA} : p_i^{(r)} < p_{i'}^{(r)}$,
(8.25)

we can use the one-sided two-sample Z-test. We consider test procedures for all-pairwise comparisons of $\{$the null hypothesis $H_{(i,i')}^{(r)}$ versus the alternative $H_{(i,i')}^{(r)OA} \mid (i, i') \in \mathcal{U}_{k^{(r)}}\}$, where $\mathcal{U}_{k^{(r)}}$ is defined by (8.3). Under the equality of sample sizes $n_1^{(r)} = \ldots = n_{k^{(r)}}^{(r)}$, corresponding to Sect. 6.3, we propose single-step simultaneous tests for $\{$the null hypothesis $H_{(i,i')}^{(r)}$ versus the alternative $H_{(i,i')}^{(r)OA} \mid (i, i') \in \mathcal{U}_{k^{(r)}}\}$.

We add the assumption (A5) of equal sample sizes.

(A5) $n_1^{(r)} = n_2^{(r)} = \ldots = n_{k^{(r)}}^{(r)} \ (r = 1, \ldots, q).$

Then $T_{i'i}^{(r)}$ of (8.8) is given by

$$T_{i'i}^{(r)} = \sqrt{2n_1^{(r)}} \left\{ \arcsin\left(\sqrt{\hat{p}_{i'}^{(r)}}\right) - \arcsin\left(\sqrt{\hat{p}_i^{(r)}}\right) \right\}. \tag{8.26}$$

We put

$$D_1(t|k^{(r)}) := P\left(\max_{1 \leq i < i' \leq k^{(r)}} \frac{Z_{i'} - Z_i}{\sqrt{2}} \leq t \right), \tag{8.27}$$

where $Z_i \sim N(0, 1) \ (i = 1, \ldots, k^{(r)})$ and $Z_1, \ldots, Z_{k^{(r)}}$ are independent. Shiraishi (2014) gives

$$\lim_{n^{(r)} \to \infty} P_{(r)0}\left(\max_{1 \leq i < i' \leq k^{(r)}} T_{i'i}^{(r)} \leq t \right) = D_1(t|k^{(r)}). \tag{8.28}$$

From Shiraishi et al. (2019), we get the following recurrence formula.

$$h_1(t, x) := P\left(\frac{Z_1 - x}{\sqrt{2}} \le t\right) = \Phi(\sqrt{2} \cdot t + x), \tag{8.29}$$

$$h_r(t, x) := \int_{-\infty}^{x} h_{r-1}(t, y)\varphi(y)dy$$
$$+ h_{r-1}(t, x)\{\Phi(\sqrt{2} \cdot t + x) - \Phi(x)\} \quad (2 \le r \le k^{(r)} - 1), \tag{8.30}$$

$$D_1(t|k^{(r)}) = \int_{-\infty}^{\infty} h_{k-1}(t, x)\varphi(x)dx. \tag{8.31}$$

For a given α such that $0 < \alpha < 1$, we put

$$d_1(k^{(r)}; \alpha) := \text{a solution of } t \text{ satisfying the equation } D_1(t|k^{(r)}) = 1 - \alpha. \tag{8.32}$$

By using (8.32), we can derive single-step procedures proposed by Hayter (1990).

[8.4] Single-Step Tests Based on One-Sided Z-Test Statistics

The asymptotic simultaneous test of level α for the {null hypothesis $H_{(i,i')}^{(r)}$ versus alternative hypothesis $H_{(i,i')}^{(r)OA} : p_i^{(r)} < p_{i'}^{(r)} \mid (i, i') \in \mathcal{U}_{k^{(r)}}$} consist in rejecting $H_{(i,i')}^{(r)}$ for $(i, i') \in \mathcal{U}_{k^{(r)}}$ such that $T_{i'i} > d_1(k^{(r)}; \alpha)$.

Next, we introduce closed testing procedures. The closure of $\mathcal{H}_1^{(r)}$ under the order restrictions (8.20) is given by

$$\overline{\mathcal{H}}_1^{(r)o} = \left\{\bigwedge_{v \in V} H_v^{(r)} \,\middle|\, \emptyset \subsetneq V \subset \mathcal{U}_{k^{(r)}}\right\} = \left\{\bigwedge_{v \in V^+} H_v^{(r)} \,\middle|\, \emptyset \subsetneq V \subset \mathcal{U}_{k^{(r)}}\right\}, \tag{8.33}$$

where
$$V^+ := \{(i, i+1)\mid \text{For } (i_0, i_0') \in V, \ i_0 \le i < i+1 \le i_0'\}. \tag{8.34}$$

Then, we get

$$\bigwedge_{v \in V} H_v^{(r)} = \bigwedge_{v \in V^+} H_v^{(r)} : \text{for any } (i, i') \in V, \ p_i^{(r)} = p_{i'}^{(r)} \text{ holds.} \tag{8.35}$$

Let $I_1^{(r)o}, \ldots, I_{J^{(r)}}^{(r)o}$ be disjoint sets satisfying the following property (P3).

(P3) There exist integers $\ell_1^{(r)}, \ldots, \ell_{J^{(r)}}^{(r)} \ge 2$ and integers $0 \le s_1^{(r)} < \ldots < s_{J^{(r)}}^{(r)} < k^{(r)}$ such that

$$I_j^{(r)o} = \{s_j^{(r)} + 1, s_j^{(r)} + 2, \ldots, s_j^{(r)} + \ell_j^{(r)}\} \ (j = 1, \ldots, J^{(r)}) \tag{8.36}$$

$$\text{and } s_j^{(r)} + \ell_j^{(r)} \le s_{j+1}^{(r)} \ (j = 1, \ldots, J^{(r)} - 1).$$

We define the null hypothesis $H^{(r)o}(I_1^{(r)o}, \ldots, I_{J^{(r)}}^{(r)o})$ by

$H^{(r)o}(I_1^{(r)o}, \ldots, I_{J^{(r)}}^{(r)o})$: for any j such that $1 \leq j \leq J^{(r)}$ and

$$\text{for any } i, i' \in I_j^{(r)o}, \ p_i^{(r)} = p_{i'}^{(r)} \text{ holds.} \tag{8.37}$$

The elements of $I_j^{(r)o}$ are consecutive integers and $\ell_j^{(r)} = \#(I_j^{(r)o}) \geq 2$. From (8.37), for any nonempty $V \subset \mathscr{U}_{k^{(r)}}$, there exist an integer $J^{(r)}$ and some subsets $I_1^{(r)o}, \ldots,$ $I_{J^{(r)}}^{(r)o} \subset \{1, \ldots, k^{(r)}\}$ satisfying (P3) such that

$$\bigwedge_{v \in V} H_v^{(r)} = \bigwedge_{v \in V^+} H_v^{(r)} = H^{(r)o}(I_1^{(r)o}, \ldots, I_{J^{(r)}}^{(r)o}). \tag{8.38}$$

Furthermore, $H^{(r)o}(I_1^{(r)o}, \ldots, I_{J^{(r)}}^{(r)o})$ is expressed as

$$H^{(r)o}(I_1^{(r)o}, \ldots, I_{J^{(r)}}^{(r)o}) : p_{s_j^{(r)}+1}^{(r)} = p_{s_j^{(r)}+2}^{(r)} = \cdots = p_{s_j^{(r)}+\ell_j^{(r)}}^{(r)} \ (j = 1, \ldots, J^{(r)}). \tag{8.39}$$

Let us put

$$T^{(r)o}(I_j^{(r)o}) := \max_{s_j^{(r)}+1 \leq i < i' \leq s_j^{(r)}+\ell_j^{(r)}} T_{i'i}^{(r)} \ (j = 1, \ldots, J^{(r)}),$$

where $I_j^{(r)o}$ is defined in (P3) and $T_{i'i}^{(r)}$ is defined by (8.26).

Corresponding to (8.28) and (8.32), for $\ell^{(r)}$ such that $2 \leq \ell^{(r)} \leq k^{(r)}$, we put

$$D_1(t|\ell^{(r)}) := P\left(\max_{1 \leq i < i' \leq \ell^{(r)}} \frac{Z_{i'} - Z_i}{\sqrt{2}} \leq t\right), \tag{8.40}$$

where Z_i's are random variables used in (8.27).

Then, we propose the stepwise procedure [8.5].

[8.5] Stepwise Procedure Based on One-Sided Z-Test Statistics
For $H^{(r)o}(I_1^{(r)o}, \ldots, I_{J^{(r)}}^{(r)o})$ of (8.38), we set

$$M^{(r)} = M^{(r)}(I_1^{(r)o}, \ldots, I_{J^{(r)}}^{(r)o}) = \sum_{j=1}^{J^{(r)}} \ell_j^{(r)}. \tag{8.41}$$

For $\ell^{(r)} = \ell_1^{(r)}, \ldots, \ell_J^{(r)}$, we define $\alpha(M^{(r)}, \ell^{(r)})$ by (8.17). By obeying the notation $d_1(\ell^{(r)}; \alpha)$, we get

$$D_1(d_1(\ell^{(r)}; \alpha(M^{(r)}, \ell^{(r)}))|\ell^{(r)}) = 1 - \alpha(M^{(r)}, \ell^{(r)}), \tag{8.42}$$

that is, $d_1(\ell^{(r)}; \alpha(M^{(r)}, \ell^{(r)}))$ is an upper $100\alpha(M^{(r)}, \ell^{(r)})\%$ point of the distribution $D_1(t|\ell^{(r)})$.

(a) $J^{(r)} \geq 2$

Whenever $d_1\left(\ell_j^{(r)}; \alpha(M^{(r)}, \ell_j^{(r)})\right) < T^{(r)o}(I_j^{(r)o})$ holds for an integer j such that $1 \leq j \leq J^{(r)}$, we reject the hypothesis $\bigwedge_{v \in V^+} H_v^{(r)}$.

(b) $J^{(r)} = 1 \; (M^{(r)} = \ell_1^{(r)})$

Whenever $d_1\left(M^{(r)}; \alpha\right) < T^{(r)o}(I_1^{(r)o})$, we reject the hypothesis $\bigwedge_{v \in V^+} H_v^{(r)}$.

By using the methods of (a) and (b), when $\bigwedge_{v \in V^+} H_v^{(r)}$ is rejected for any V such that $(i, i') \in V \subset \mathcal{U}_{k^{(r)}}$, the null hypothesis $H_{(i,i')}^{(r)}$ is rejected as a multiple comparison test, where V^+ is defined by (8.34).

We do not impose the assumption (A5) of equal sample sizes from now on. The discussions of (8.33)–(8.39) do not depend on (A5).

For $I_j^{(r)o}$ of (8.36) and $j = 1, \ldots, J^{(r)}$, we define $\hat{v}_{s_j^{(r)}+1}^{(r)o}(I_j^{(r)o}), \ldots, \hat{v}_{s_j^{(r)}+\ell_j^{(r)}}^{(r)o}(I_j^{(r)o})$

by $u_{s_j^{(r)}+1}, \ldots, u_{s_j^{(r)}+\ell_j^{(r)}}$ which minimize $\sum_{i \in I_j^{(r)o}} \lambda_{ni}^{(r)}\left(u_i - \hat{v}_i^{(r)}\right)^2$ under simple order restrictions $u_{s_j^{(r)}+1} \leq u_{s_j^{(r)}+2} \leq \cdots \leq u_{s_j^{(r)}+\ell_j^{(r)}}$, i.e.,

$$\sum_{i \in I_j^{(r)o}} \lambda_{ni}^{(r)}\left(\hat{v}_i^{(r)o}(I_j^{(r)o}) - \hat{v}_i^{(r)}\right)^2 = \min_{u_{s_j^{(r)}+1} \leq \cdots \leq u_{s_j^{(r)}+\ell_j^{(r)}}} \sum_{i \in I_j^{(r)o}} \lambda_{ni}^{(r)}\left(u_i - \hat{v}_i^{(r)}\right)^2.$$

Corresponding to (8.22), we get

$$\hat{v}_{s_j^{(r)}+m}^{(r)o}(I_j^{(r)o}) = \max_{s_j^{(r)}+1 \leq a \leq s_j^{(r)}+m} \;\; \min_{s_j^{(r)}+m \leq b \leq s_j^{(r)}+\ell_j^{(r)}} \;\; \frac{\sum_{i=a}^{b} n_i^{(r)}\hat{v}_i^{(r)}}{\sum_{i=a}^{b} n_i^{(r)}} \quad (m = 1, \ldots, \ell_j^{(r)}).$$

We put

$$\bar{\chi}_{\ell_j^{(r)}}^2(I_j^{(r)o}) := \sum_{i \in I_j^{(r)o}} n_i^{(r)}\left(\hat{v}_i^{(r)o}(I_j^{(r)o}) - \sum_{i \in I_j^{(r)o}}\left(\frac{n_i^{(r)}}{n^{(r)}(I_j^{(r)o})}\right)\hat{v}_i^{(r)}\right)^2, \qquad (8.43)$$

where

$$n^{(r)}(I_j^{(r)o}) := \sum_{i \in I_j^{(r)o}} n_i^{(r)}.$$

We define $\breve{v}_1^{(r)o}, \ldots, \breve{v}_{\ell_j^{(r)}}^{(r)o}$ by

$$\sum_{i=1}^{\ell_j^{(r)}} \lambda_{s_j^{(r)}+i}^{(r)}\left(\breve{v}_i^{(r)o} - Z_i\right)^2 = \min_{u_1 \leq \cdots \leq u_{\ell_j^{(r)}}} \sum_{i=1}^{\ell_j^{(r)}} \lambda_{s_j^{(r)}+i}^{(r)}(u_i - Z_i)^2$$

where $Z_1, \ldots, Z_{\ell_j^{(r)}}$ are independent and $Z_i \sim N(0, 1/\lambda_{s_j^{(r)}+i}^{(r)})$ $(i = 1, \ldots, \ell_j^{(r)})$. Let $P(L, \ell_j^{(r)}; \lambda^{(r)}(I_j^{(r)o}))$ be the probability that $\breve{v}_1^{(r)o}, \ldots, \breve{v}_{\ell_j^{(r)}}^{(r)o}$ takes exactly L distinct values, where $\lambda^{(r)}(I_j^{(r)o}) := (\lambda_{s_j^{(r)}+1}^{(r)}, \ldots, \lambda_{s_j^{(r)}+\ell_j^{(r)}}^{(r)})$. Then, for $t > 0$, under the condition (A4), we get

$$
\lim_{n^{(r)} \to \infty} P_{(r)0} \left(\bar{\chi}_{\ell_j^{(r)}}^2(I_j^{(r)o}) \geq t \right) = \sum_{L=2}^{\ell_j^{(r)}} P(L, \ell_j^{(r)}; \lambda^{(r)}(I_j^{(r)o})) P \left(\chi_{L-1}^2 \geq t \right). \quad (8.44)
$$

For a given α such that $0 < \alpha < 0.5$, we put

$$
\bar{c}^2 \left(\ell_j^{(r)}, \lambda^{(r)}(I_j^{(r)o}); \alpha \right) := \text{a solution of } t \text{ satisfying the equation}
$$

$$
\sum_{L=2}^{\ell_j^{(r)}} P(L, \ell_j^{(r)}; \lambda^{(r)}(I_j^{(r)o})) P \left(\chi_{L-1}^2 \geq t \right) = \alpha. \quad (8.45)
$$

Then, we propose the stepwise procedure [8.6].

[8.6] Stepwise Procedure Based on $\bar{\chi}^2$-Statistics
For $H^{(r)o}(I_1^{(r)o}, \ldots, I_{J^{(r)}}^{(r)o})$ of (8.38) and for $\ell^{(r)} = \ell_1^{(r)}, \ldots, \ell_J^{(r)}$, we define $M^{(r)}$ and $\alpha(M^{(r)}, \ell^{(r)})$ by (8.41) and (8.17), respectively.

(a) $J^{(r)} \geq 2$
    Whenever $\bar{c}^2 \left(\ell_j^{(r)}, \lambda^{(r)}(I_j^{(r)o}); \alpha(M^{(r)}, \ell_j^{(r)}) \right) < \bar{\chi}_{\ell_j^{(r)}}^2(I_j^{(r)o})$ holds for an integer j such that $1 \leq j \leq J$, we reject the hypothesis $\bigwedge_{v \in V+} H_v^{(r)}$.
(b) $J^{(r)} = 1$ $(M^{(r)} = \ell_1^{(r)})$
    Whenever $\bar{c}^2 \left(\ell_1^{(r)}, \lambda^{(r)}(I_1^{(r)o}); \alpha \right) < \bar{\chi}_{\ell_1^{(r)}}^2(I_1^{(r)o})$, we reject the hypothesis $\bigwedge_{v \in V+} H_v^{(r)}$.

By using the methods of (a) and (b), when $\bigwedge_{v \in V+} H_v^{(r)}$ is rejected for any V such that $(i, i') \in V \subset \mathcal{U}_{k^{(r)}}$, the null hypothesis $H_{(i,i')}^{(r)}$ is rejected as a multiple comparison test, where V^+ is defined by (8.34).

8.4 Serial Gatekeeping Procedures

Suppose that the families $\mathcal{H}_1^{(1)}, \ldots, \mathcal{H}_1^{(q)}$ of null hypotheses has the order (8.4) of priority. Furthermore, suppose that, for some r, simple order restrictions $p_1^{(r)} \leq p_2^{(r)} \leq \ldots \leq p_{k^{(r)}}^{(r)}$ hold. Let us put the set

$$
O_q := \{r \mid p_1^{(r)} \leq p_2^{(r)} \leq \ldots \leq p_{k^{(r)}}^{(r)} \text{ is satisfied and } 1 \leq r \leq q\}. \quad (8.46)
$$

Then we propose multiple test procedures for all-pairwise comparisons of

$$\{\text{the null hypothesis } H_{(i,i')}^{(r)} \text{ versus the alternative}$$

$$H_{(i,i')}^{(r)A} \text{ or } H_{(i,i')}^{(r)OA} \big| (i,i') \in \mathcal{U}_{k^{(r)}}, \ 1 \le r \le q\}, \qquad (8.47)$$

where we choose $H_{(i,i')}^{(r)A}$ as the alternative hypothesis for $r \in O_q^c \cap \{1, \ldots, q\}$ and choose $H_{(i,i')}^{(r)OA}$ for $r \in O_q$. In Sects. 8.1 and 8.2, we state multiple tests among $p_1^{(r)}, \ldots, p_{k^{(r)}}^{(r)}$ for fixed r. In this section, we discuss multiple tests among $p_1^{(r)}, \ldots, p_{k^{(r)}}^{(r)}$ for all r's. Corresponding to (A4), we add the assumption of

$$(A6) \qquad \lim_{n^{(r)} \to \infty} \frac{n_i^{(r)}}{n^{(r)}} = \lambda_i^{(r)} > 0, \quad (1 \le i \le k^{(r)}, \ 1 \le r \le q).$$

Since the serial gatekeeping procedures are closed testing procedures, we introduce closed testing procedures for $\bigcup_{r=1}^{q} \mathcal{H}_1^{(r)}$.

The closure of $\bigcup_{r=1}^{q} \mathcal{H}_1^{(r)}$ is given by

$$\overline{\bigcup_{r=1}^{q} \mathcal{H}_1^{(r)}} \equiv \left\{ \bigwedge_{g=1}^{h} \left(\bigwedge_{v \in V^{(r_g)}} H_v^{(r_g)} \right) \, \middle| \, \text{there exist integer } h \text{ and integers } r_1, \ldots, r_h \right.$$

$$\text{such that } 1 \le h \le q, \ 1 \le r_1 < \ldots < r_h \le q, \text{ and}$$

$$\left. \emptyset \subsetneq V^{(r_g)} \subset \mathcal{U}_{k^{(r_g)}} \ (1 \le g \le h) \text{ hold} \right\}.$$

Then, we get

$$\bigwedge_{g=1}^{h} \left(\bigwedge_{v \in V^{(r_g)}} H_v^{(r_g)} \right) : \text{for any } g \text{ such that } 1 \le g \le h \text{ and for any } (i,i') \in V^{(r_g)},$$

$$p_i^{(r_g)} = p_{i'}^{(r_g)} \text{ holds}.$$

Then, from (8.15) and (8.38), for any nonempty $V^{(r_g)} \subset \mathcal{U}_{k^{(r_g)}}$, there exist an integer $J^{(r_g)}$ and disjoint sets $I_1^{(r_g)*}, \ldots, I_{J^{(r_g)}}^{(r_g)*}$ such that

$$\bigwedge_{v \in V^{(r_g)}} H_v^{(r_g)} = H^{(r_g)*}(I_1^{(r_g)*}, \ldots, I_{J^{(r_g)}}^{(r_g)*}) \qquad (8.48)$$

and $\#(I_j^{(r_g)*}) \ge 2 \ (j = 1, \ldots, J^{(r_g)})$,

where $H^{(r_g)*}(I_1^{(r_g)*}, \ldots, I_{J^{(r_g)}}^{(r_g)*})$ stands for

$$H^{(r_g)*}(I_1^{(r_g)*}, \ldots, I_{J^{(r_g)}}^{(r_g)*}) := \begin{cases} H^{(r_g)}(I_1^{(r_g)}, \ldots, I_{J^{(r_g)}}^{(r_g)}) & (r_g \in O_q^c \cap \{1, \ldots, q\}) \\ H^{(r_g)o}(I_1^{(r_g)o}, \ldots, I_{J^{(r_g)}}^{(r_g)o}) & (r_g \in O_q), \end{cases}$$

and, for $j = 1, \ldots, J_{r_g}$, $I_j^{(r_g)*}$ stands for

$$I_j^{(r_g)*} := \begin{cases} I_j^{(r_g)} & (r_g \in O_q^c \cap \{1, \ldots, q\}) \\ I_j^{(r_g)o} & (r_g \in O_q). \end{cases}$$

Hence, we get

$$\bigwedge_{g=1}^{h} \left(\bigwedge_{v \in V^{(r_g)}} H_v^{(r_g)} \right) = \bigwedge_{g=1}^{h} H^{(r_g)*}(I_1^{(r_g)*}, \ldots, I_{J^{(r_g)}}^{(r_g)*}), \tag{8.49}$$

where $1 \le r_1 < \ldots < r_h \le q$.

[8.7] Hybrid Serial Gatekeeping Procedures

For integer r such that $1 \le r \le q$, in ascending order, perform multiple comparison test of level α based on stepwise procedure [8.3] or [8.6], where we choose [8.3] for $r \in O_q^c \cap \{1, \ldots, q\}$ and choose [8.6] for $r \in O_q$. Then we reject null hypotheses in $\bigcup_{r=1}^{q} \mathcal{H}_1^{(r)}$ obeying the following (b1)-(b3).

(b1) When there is a null hypothesis in $\mathcal{H}_1^{(1)}$ that is not rejected by the stepwise procedure [8.3] or [8.6], only the null hypothesis rejected in $\mathcal{H}_1^{(1)}$ is rejected as a multiple comparison test.

(b2) When there exists an integer q_0 satisfying $q_0 < q$ that, for any r such that $1 \le r \le q_0$, all the null hypotheses in $\mathcal{H}_1^{(r)}$ are rejected by stepwise procedure [8.3] or [8.6] and there is a null hypothesis in $\mathcal{H}_1^{(q_0+1)}$ that is not rejected, all the null hypotheses in $\bigcup_{r=1}^{q_0} \mathcal{H}_1^{(r)}$ are rejected as a multiple comparison test and only the null hypothesis rejected in $\mathcal{H}_1^{(q_0+1)}$ is rejected.

(b3) When, for any r satisfying $1 \le r \le q$, all the null hypotheses in $\mathcal{H}_1^{(r)}$ are rejected by stepwise procedure [8.3] or [8.6], all the null hypotheses in $\bigcup_{r=1}^{q} \mathcal{H}_1^{(r)}$ are rejected as a multiple comparison test.

Theorem 8.1 *Suppose that the assumption (A6) is satisfied. Then the test procedure [8.7] is an asymptotic multiple comparison test of level α.*

Proof It is enough to show that [8.7] is a closed testing procedure of level α.
The test of level α for $H^{(r_1)*}(I_1^{(r_1)*}, \ldots, I_{J^{(r_1)}}^{(r_1)*})$ is executed. Furthermore, when $h \ge 2$ in (8.49), the test of level 0 for $H^{(r_g)*}(I_1^{(r_g)*}, \ldots, I_{J^{(r_g)}}^{(r_g)*})$ is executed for any g such that $2 \le g \le h$. As these results, we are able to decide whether or not the hypothesis $\bigwedge_{g=1}^{h} \left(\bigwedge_{v \in V^{(r_g)}} H_v^{(r_g)} \right)$ is rejected. Let us refer to this method as A-procedure.

(1). The case of (b1)

Suppose that $H_{(i_1,i_1')}^{(1)}$ is rejected by using the procedure [8.7]. Then, from A-procedure, $r_1 = 1$ holds and there exists j such that all the null hypotheses (8.49) satisfying i_1, $i_1' \in I_j^{(1)*}$ and $1 \leq j \leq J^{(1)}$ are rejected. Suppose that $H_{(i_2,i_2')}^{(1)}$ is not rejected by using the procedure [8.7]. Then, from A-procedure, $r_1 = 1$ holds and there exists j' such that some null hypothesis (8.48) satisfying i_2, $i_2' \in I_{j'}^{(1)*}$ and $1 \leq j' \leq J^{(1)}$ is not rejected. Let $H^{(1)*}(I_{01}^{(1)*}, \ldots, I_{0J^{(1)}}^{(1)*})$ be the null hypothesis that is not rejected. Then, from A-procedure, $H_{(i_2,i_2')}^{(1)}$ is not rejected.

From A-procedure, $H^{(1)*}(I_{01}^{(1)*}, \ldots, I_{0J^{(1)}}^{(1)*}) \bigwedge \left(\bigwedge_{g=2}^h H^{(r_g)*}(I_1^{(r_g)*}, \ldots, I_{J^{(r_g)}}^{(r_g)*}) \right)$

is not rejected. Therefore, all the null hypotheses in $\bigcup_{r=2}^q \mathscr{H}_1^{(r)}$ are not rejected.

(2). The case of (b2)

Since any null hypothesis (8.49) satisfying $1 \leq r_1 \leq q_0$ is rejected, for any r such that $1 \leq r \leq q_0$, all the null hypotheses in $\mathscr{H}_1^{(r)}$ are rejected. Suppose that $H_{(i_1,i_1')}^{(q_0+1)}$ in $\mathscr{H}_1^{(q_0+1)}$ is rejected by using the procedure [8.7]. Then, from A-procedure, $r_1 = q_0 + 1$ holds and there exists j such that all the null hypotheses (8.49) satisfying i_1, $i_1' \in I_j^{(q_0+1)*}$ and $1 \leq j \leq J^{(q_0)}$ are rejected. Suppose that $H_{(i_2,i_2')}^{(q_0+1)}$ in $\mathscr{H}_1^{(q_0+1)}$ is not rejected by using the procedure [8.7]. Then, from A-procedure, $r_1 = q_0 + 1$ holds and there exists j' such that some null hypothesis (8.48) satisfying i_2, $i_2' \in I_{j'}^{(q_0+1)*}$ and $1 \leq j' \leq J^{(q_0+1)}$ is not rejected. Let $H^{(q_0+1)*}(I_{01}^{(q_0+1)*}, \ldots, I_{0J^{(q_0+1)}}^{(q_0+1)*})$ be the null hypothesis that is not rejected. Then, from A-procedure, $H_{(i_2,i_2')}^{(q_0+1)}$ is not rejected. From A-procedure,

$$H^{(q_0+1)*}(I_{01}^{(q_0+1)*}, \ldots, I_{0J^{(q_0+1)}}^{(q_0+1)*}) \bigwedge \left(\bigwedge_{g=2}^h H^{(r_g)*}(I_1^{(r_g)*}, \ldots, I_{J^{(r_g)}}^{(r_g)*}) \right) \quad (q_0 + 1$$

$< r_2)$ is not rejected. Therefore, all the null hypotheses in $\bigcup_{r=q_0+2}^q \mathscr{H}_1^{(r)}$ are not rejected.

(3) The case of (b3)

From A-procedure, it is self-evident that all the null hypotheses in $\left\{ H_{(i,i')}^{(r)} \mid (i, i') \in \mathscr{U}_{k^{(r)}}, \ 1 \leq r \leq q \right\}$ are rejected.

From (1)–(3), the closed testing procedure of level α for (9.26) based on A-procedure is equivalent to the procedure [8.7]. $\square$

Even if we replace [8.3] with [8.1] or [8.2] in the hybrid serial gatekeeping procedures [8.7], Theorem 8.1 still holds. Furthermore, even if we replace [8.6] with [8.4] or [8.5] in [8.7], Theorem 8.1 still holds under the condition (A4) of equal sample sizes.

8.5   Application to Multivariate Multi-sample Models

Let $\{X_{ij} = (X_{ij}^{(1)}, \ldots, X_{ij}^{(q)})^T \mid j = 1, \ldots, n_i, \ i = 1, \ldots, k\}$ be a set of independent vector-valued random variables. Then $\left(X_{i1}^{(r)}, \ldots, X_{in_i}^{(r)}\right)$ is a random sample of size n_i from the i-th Bernoulli population with success probability $p_i^{(r)}$ $(i = 1, \ldots, k,$ $r = 1, \ldots, q)$. It is convenient to assign the number 1 to a success and the number 0 to a failure.

$$P(X_{ij}^{(r)} = 1) = p_i^{(r)} \text{ and } P(X_{ij}^{(r)} = 0) = 1 - p_i^{(r)}$$

hold. $X_{i1}^{(r)}, \ldots, X_{in_i}^{(r)}$ are assumed to be independent. We need not assume that $X^{(1)}, \ldots, X^{(q)}$ are independent, where $X^{(r)} := \left(X_{11}^{(r)}, \ldots, X_{kn_k}^{(r)}\right)$. Furthermore, the model is limited to

$$k^{(r)} = k \ (r = 1, \ldots, q) \text{ and } n_i^{(r)} = n_i \ (i = 1, \ldots, k, \ r = 1, \ldots, q). \qquad (8.50)$$

The notations of $\mathcal{U}_{k^{(r)}}$ and $n^{(r)}$ are simplified to

$$\mathcal{U}_{k^{(r)}} = \mathcal{U}_k = \{(i, i') \mid 1 \le i < i' \le k\} \text{ and } n^{(r)} = n = \sum_{i=1}^{k} n_i.$$

In the q variate k-sample model, gatekeeping procedures [8.7] give multiple comparison tests of level α for all-pairwise comparisons of

$$\left\{\text{the null hypothesis } H_{(i,i')}^{(r)} \text{ versus the alternative}\right.$$
$$\left. H_{(i,i')}^{(r)A} \text{ or } H_{(i,i')}^{(r)OA} \middle| (i, i') \in \mathcal{U}_k, \ 1 \le r \le q\right\}$$

under the limits of (8.50).

8.6   Discussion

When the families of null hypotheses $\mathcal{F}_r = \{H_{pj} \mid j = 1, \ldots, m_r\}$ $(r = 1, \ldots, q)$ have the order of priority, $\mathcal{F}_1 \succ \ldots \succ \mathcal{F}_q$, Mauer (1995) proposed a multiple comparison test using a closed test procedure called the serial gatekeeping method. The serial gatekeeping procedures are based on Bonferroni tests and the test procedure of Holm (1979). In the serial gatekeeping method, the tests are performed in the order of the null hypothesis family $\mathcal{F}_1, \ldots, \mathcal{F}_q$. If a null hypothesis in the $\mathcal{F}_r$ $(1 \le r < q)$ is not rejected, test procedures for the subsequent null hypothesis family $\mathcal{F}_{r+1}, \ldots, \mathcal{F}_q$ are not performed. As a closed test procedure that covers this shortcoming, Dmitrienko et al. (2003) proposed a multiple comparison test called the parallel gatekeeping procedure. In the parallel gatekeeping procedure, Bonferroni's method is used. Since the parallel gatekeeping procedure is not simple, it is difficult to propose the parallel gatekeeping procedure based on [8.1]–[8.6] as a multiple comparison test of level α. It is simple to use the hybrid serial gatekeeping procedure by replacing [8.3] and [8.6] with [8.1] and [8.4], respectively in [8.7]. Under simple order restrictions of (8.20), Shiraishi and Matsuda (2016) investigate the all-pairs power proposed by Ramsey (1978) for $q = 1$. As a result, the order of the power is following:

$$[8.6] \geq [8.5] > [8.3] \geq [8.2] > [8.4] > [8.1]. \tag{8.51}$$

In the all-pairs power of specified alternatives, [8.6] is a little superior to [8.5], and [8.3] is a little superior to [8.2].

We suppose the reverse order restrictions

$$p_1^{(r)} \geq p_2^{(r)} \geq \cdots \geq p_{k^{(r)}}^{(r)}. \tag{8.52}$$

Then we put $Y_{ij}^{(r)} := 1 - X_{ij}^{(r)}$ $(j = 1, \ldots n_i^{(r)}; \ i = 1, \ldots, k^{(r)})$. $(Y_{i1}^{(r)}, \ldots, Y_{in_i^{(r)}}^{(r)})$ is a random sample of size $n_i^{(r)}$ from the i-th normal population with unknown mean $p_i'^{(r)} = 1 - p_i^{(r)}$ $(i = 1, \ldots, k^{(r)})$ and unknown variance $\sigma_{(r)}^2$. Equation (8.52) is equivalent to the simple order restrictions of $p_i'^{(r)}$'s: $p_1'^{(r)} \leq p_2'^{(r)} \leq \cdots \leq p_{k^{(r)}}'^{(r)}$. By replacing $X_{ij}^{(r)}$ with $Y_{ij}^{(r)}$ in all statistics of Sects. 8.2 and 8.3, we can discuss the multiple comparison procedures under the restrictions (8.52).

References

Barlow RE, Bartholomew DJ, Bremner JM, Brunk HD (1972) Statistical inference under order restrictions. Wiley, London

Dmitrienko A, Offen W, Westfall PH (2003) Gatekeeping strategies for clinical trials that do not require all primary effects to be significant. Stat Med 22:2387–2400

Enderton HB (2001) A mathematical introduction to logic, 2nd edn. Academic, New York

Hayter AJ (1984) A proof of the conjecture that the Tukey-Kramer multiple comparisons procedure is conservative. Ann Stat 12:61–75

Hayter AJ (1990) A one-sided studentized range test for testing against a simple ordered alternative. J Amer Statist Assoc 85:778–785

Lund J, Bowers KL (1992) Sinc methods for quadrature and differential equations. Siam

Maurer W, Hothorn L, Lehmacher W (1995) Multiple comparisons in drug clinical trials and preclinical assays: a priori ordered hypotheses. In Biometrie in der ChemischPharmazeutischen Industrie 6:3–18

Ramsey PH (1978) Power differences between pairwise multiple comparisons. J Amer Statist Assoc 73:479–485

Robertson T, Wright FT, Dykstra RL (1988) Order restricted statistical inference. Wiley, London

Shiraishi T (2006) The upper bound for the distribution of Tukey-Kramer's statistic. Bull Comput Stat 19:77–87 (in Japanese)

Shiraishi T (2014) Closed testing procedures in multi-sample models under a simple ordered restriction. J Japan Statist Soc 43:215–245 (in Japanese)

Shiraishi T, Sugiura H (2015) The upper $100\alpha^\star$th percentiles of the distributions used in multiple comparison procedures under a simple order restriction. J Japan Stat Soc Japanese Issue 44:271–314 (in Japanese)

Shiraishi T, Sugiura H (2018) Theory of multiple comparison procedures and its computation. Kyoritsu-Shuppan Co., Ltd. (in Japanese)

Shiraishi T, Sugiura H, Matsuda S (2019) Pairwise multiple comparisons-theory and computation. Springer

Stenger F (1993) Numerical methods based on Sinc and analytic function. Springer-Verlag

Westfall PH, Krishen A (2001) Optimally weighted, fixed sequence and gatekeeper multiple testing procedures. J Stat Plan Inference 99:25–41

Williams DA (1971) A test for differences between treatment means when several dose levels are compared with a zero dose control. Biometrics 27:103–117

Chapter 9
Hybrid Serial Gatekeeping Procedures for Multiple Comparisons with a Control

Abstract In q multi-sample models, we consider multiple comparison tests with a control. Let $\mathcal{H}_2^{(r)}$ be the family of null hypothesis among $k^{(r)}$ proportions for $r = 1, \ldots, q$. The family $\mathcal{H}_2^{(1)} \succ \ldots \succ \mathcal{H}_2^{(q)}$ has the order of priority. This chapter describes procedures for performing multiple comparison tests at level α based on serial gatekeeping methods. In the r-th stage, a test procedure under unrestricted proportions or a test procedure under order restricted proportions is used. The proposed hybrid procedures are the methods assuming the Bernoulli distribution. The power of the proposed tests is much superior to the serial gatekeeping methods based on Bonferroni tests which are proposed by Mauer et al. (1995).

9.1 Introduction

We consider k-sample models with Bernoulli responses. $(X_{i1}, \ldots, X_{in_i})$ is a random sample of size n_i from the i-th Bernoulli population with success probability p_i $(i = 1, \ldots, k)$. It is convenient to assign the number 1 to a success and the number 0 to a failure.

$$P(X_{ij} = 1) = p_i \text{ and } P(X_{ij} = 0) = 1 - p_i$$

hold. X_{ij}'s are assumed to be independent. Suppose that p_1 is the proportion of the control and $p_2, \ldots, p_k$ are the proportions of the new treatments. Chapter 4 discussed Dunnett-type single-step procedures [4.1] as three multiple comparisons with a control for $\{$the null hypothesis $H_i : p_i = p_1$ vs. the alternative $H_i^{A\pm} : p_i \neq p_1 | i \in \mathcal{I}_{2,k}\}$, $\{$the null hypothesis H_i vs. the alternative $H_i^{A+} : p_i > p_1 | i \in \mathcal{I}_{2,k}\}$, and $\{$the null hypothesis H_i vs. the alternative $H_i^{A-} : p_i < p_1 | i \in \mathcal{I}_{2,k}\}$, where $\mathcal{I}_{2,k} := \{i \mid 2 \leq i \leq k\}$.

When the simple order restrictions

$$p_1 \leq p_2 \leq \ldots \leq p_k$$

are satisfied, Chap. 7 stated Williams-type multi-step tests for {the null hypothesis H_i vs. the alternative $H_i^{A+} : p_i > p_1 \big| i \in \mathscr{I}_{2,k}$} under the equal sample sizes of $n_2 = \ldots = n_k$. Chapter 7 also discussed multi-step tests based on $\bar{\chi}^2$-statistics without assuming these equal sample sizes.

Gatekeeping procedures became to be used in recent years as a convenient way to handle relationships between multiple hierarchical objectives. To solve questions concerning different objectives, null hypotheses are divided into q ordered families, $\mathscr{F}^{(1)} \succ \ldots \succ \mathscr{F}^{(q)}$. Westfall and Krishen (2001) proposed the serial gatekeeping procedures in which the hypotheses in $\mathscr{F}^{(r+1)}$ are tested if and only if all hypotheses in $\mathscr{F}^{(r)}$ are rejected ($1 \le r \le q - 1$). The individual test procedures are based on Bonferroni tests.

In this chapter, we consider q multi-sample models. In the r-th multi-sample models, $\left(X_{i1}^{(r)}, \ldots, X_{in_i^{(r)}}^{(r)} \right)$ is a random sample of size $n_i^{(r)}$ from the i-th Bernoulli population with success probability $p_i^{(r)}$ ($i = 1, \ldots, k^{(r)}$). It is convenient to assign the number 1 to a success and the number 0 to a failure.

$$P(X_{ij}^{(r)} = 1) = p_i^{(r)} \text{ and } P(X_{ij}^{(r)} = 0) = 1 - p_i^{(r)}$$

hold. $X_{i1}^{(r)}, \ldots, X_{in_i^{(r)}}^{(r)}$ are assumed to be independent. We need not assume that $X^{(1)}, \ldots, X^{(q)}$ are independent, where $X^{(r)} := \left(X_{11}^{(r)}, \ldots, X_{k^{(r)}n_{k^{(r)}}^{(r)}}^{(r)} \right)$. Let

$$\mathscr{H}_2^{(r)} := \left\{ H_i^{(r)} : p_i^{(r)} = p_1^{(r)} \big| i \in \mathscr{I}_{2,k^{(r)}} \right\} \tag{9.1}$$

be the family of null hypothesis among $k^{(r)}$ proportions for $r = 1, \ldots, q$, where

$$\mathscr{I}_{2,k^{(r)}} := \{ i \mid 2 \le i \le k^{(r)} \}. \tag{9.2}$$

The family $\mathscr{H}_2^{(1)}, \ldots, \mathscr{H}_2^{(q)}$ has the order of priority.

$$\mathscr{H}_2^{(1)} \succ \ldots \succ \mathscr{H}_2^{(q)}. \tag{9.3}$$

This paper describes procedures for performing multiple comparison tests at level α based on serial gatekeeping methods. In the r-th stage, a test procedure under unrestricted proportions or a test procedure under order restricted proportions is used. The methods of procedures [4.1], [4.2], [4.3], [7.1], and [7.2] stated in Chaps. 4 and 7 are used in the hybrid gatekeeping procedures. The power of the proposed tests is much superior to the serial gatekeeping methods based on Bonferroni tests which are usually used.

Throughout this chapter, we suppose that the assumption of (A1) stated in Sect. 3.1 is satisfied.

9.2 Multiple Comparisons Under Unrestricted Proportions in the r-th Multi-sample Model

For specified i such that $2 \leq i \leq k^{(r)}$, we are interested in testing the null hypothesis $H_i^{(r)} : p_i^{(r)} = p_1^{(r)}$. We can use the two-sided two-sample tests. In this section, we consider test procedures for comparisons of

$$\left\{ \text{the null hypothesis } H_i^{(r)} \text{ vs. the alternative } H_i^{(r)A\pm} : p_i^{(r)} \neq p_1^{(r)} \middle| i \in \mathscr{I}_{2,k^{(r)}} \right\} \tag{9.4}$$

and

$$\left\{ \text{the null hypothesis } H_i^{(r)} \text{ vs. the alternative } H_i^{(r)A+} : p_i^{(r)} > p_1^{(r)} \middle| i \in \mathscr{I}_{2,k^{(r)}} \right\}, \tag{9.5}$$

where $\mathscr{I}_{2,k^{(r)}}$ is defined by (9.2). We add the assumption of

$$(A4) \qquad \lim_{n^{(r)} \to \infty} \frac{n_i^{(r)}}{n^{(r)}} = \lambda_i^{(r)} > 0, \quad (1 \leq i \leq k^{(r)}),$$

where $n^{(r)} := \sum_{i=1}^{k} n_i^{(r)}$. We introduce two distribution functions of $B_1(t|k^{(r)}, \boldsymbol{\lambda}^{(r)})$ and $B_2(t|k^{(r)}, \boldsymbol{\lambda}^{(r)})$.

$$B_1(t|k^{(r)}, \boldsymbol{\lambda}^{(r)}) := \int_{-\infty}^{\infty} \prod_{i=2}^{k^{(r)}} \left\{ \Phi\left(\sqrt{\frac{\lambda_i^{(r)}}{\lambda_1^{(r)}}} \cdot x + \sqrt{\frac{\lambda_i^{(r)} + \lambda_1^{(r)}}{\lambda_1^{(r)}}} \cdot t \right) \right.$$
$$\left. - \Phi\left(\sqrt{\frac{\lambda_i^{(r)}}{\lambda_1^{(r)}}} \cdot x - \sqrt{\frac{\lambda_i^{(r)} + \lambda_1^{(r)}}{\lambda_1^{(r)}}} \cdot t \right) \right\} d\Phi(x),$$

$$B_2(t|k^{(r)}, \boldsymbol{\lambda}^{(r)}) := \int_{-\infty}^{\infty} \prod_{i=2}^{k^{(r)}} \Phi\left(\sqrt{\frac{\lambda_i^{(r)}}{\lambda_1^{(r)}}} \cdot x + \sqrt{\frac{\lambda_i^{(r)} + \lambda_1^{(r)}}{\lambda_1^{(r)}}} \cdot t \right) d\Phi(x),$$

where

$$\boldsymbol{\lambda}^{(r)} := (\lambda_1^{(r)}, \ldots, \lambda_{k^{(r)}}^{(r)}) \quad (r = 1, \ldots, q). \tag{9.6}$$

We put

$$T_i^{(r)} := \frac{2\left\{ \arcsin\left(\sqrt{\hat{p}_i^{(r)}}\right) - \arcsin\left(\sqrt{\hat{p}_1^{(r)}}\right) \right\}}{\sqrt{\frac{1}{n_i^{(r)}} + \frac{1}{n_1^{(r)}}}}, \quad (i \in \mathscr{I}_{2,k^{(r)}}), \tag{9.7}$$

where

$$\hat{p}_i^{(r)} := \frac{X_{i\cdot}^{(r)}}{n_i^{(r)}} \quad \text{or} \quad \frac{X_{i\cdot}^{(r)} + 0.5}{n_i^{(r)} + 1} \tag{9.8}$$

and $X_{i\cdot}^{(r)} := \sum_{j=1}^{n_i^{(r)}} X_{ij}^{(r)}$. Then, from (4.7) and (4.8) of Theorem 4.1, we get, for $t > 0$,

$$\lim_{n^{(r)} \to \infty} P_{(r)0} \left(\max_{i \in \mathscr{I}_{2,k^{(r)}}} |T_i^{(r)}| \leq t \right) = B_1(t|k^{(r)}, \boldsymbol{\lambda}^{(r)}), \tag{9.9}$$

$$\lim_{n^{(r)} \to \infty} P_{(r)0} \left(\max_{i \in \mathscr{I}_{2,k^{(r)}}} T_i^{(r)} \leq t \right) = B_2(t|k^{(r)}, \boldsymbol{\lambda}^{(r)}) \tag{9.10}$$

hold, where $P_{(r)0}(\cdot)$ stands for probability measure under the following null hypothesis $H_0^{(r)}$.

$$H_0^{(r)} : \ p_1^{(r)} = \ldots = p_{k^{(r)}}^{(r)}. \tag{9.11}$$

For a given α such that $0 < \alpha < 1$, we put

$$b_1(k^{(r)}, \lambda_1^{(r)}, \cdots, \lambda_{k^{(r)}}^{(r)}; \alpha)$$
:= a solution of t satisfying the equation $B_1(t|k^{(r)}, \boldsymbol{\lambda}^{(r)}) = 1 - \alpha$, $\quad$ (9.12)

$$b_2(k^{(r)}, \lambda_1^{(r)}, \cdots, \lambda_{k^{(r)}}^{(r)}; \alpha)$$
:= a solution of t satisfying the equation $B_2(t|k^{(r)}, \boldsymbol{\lambda}^{(r)}) = 1 - \alpha$. $\quad$ (9.13)

From (9.9) and (9.10), we get asymptotic simultaneous tests of [9.1].

[9.1] Dunnett-Type Single-Step Tests for The Alternative Hypothesis of $H_i^{(r)A\pm}$
The Dunnett-type test of level α for {the null hypothesis $H_i^{(r)}$ vs. the alternative $H_i^{(r)A\pm}\big| \ i \in \mathscr{I}_{2,k^{(r)}}$} consists in rejecting $H_i^{(r)}$ for $i \in \mathscr{I}_{2,k^{(r)}}$ such that $|T_i^{(r)}| > b_1(k^{(r)}, \lambda_1^{(r)}, \cdots, \lambda_{k^{(r)}}^{(r)}; \alpha)$.

[9.2] Dunnett-Type Single-Step Tests for the Alternative Hypothesis of $H_i^{(r)A+}$
The Dunnett-type test of level α for {the null hypothesis $H_i^{(r)}$ vs. the alternative $H_i^{(r)A+}\big| \ i \in \mathscr{I}_{2,k^{(r)}}$} consists in rejecting $H_i^{(r)}$ for $i \in \mathscr{I}_{2,k^{(r)}}$ such that $T_i^{(r)} > b_2(k^{(r)}, \lambda_1^{(r)}, \cdots, \lambda_{k^{(r)}}^{(r)}; \alpha)$.

The closure of $\mathscr{H}_2^{(r)}$ is given by

$$\overline{\mathscr{H}}_2^{(r)} := \left\{ \bigwedge_{i \in E^{(r)}} H_i^{(r)} \ \bigg| \ \emptyset \subsetneq E^{(r)} \subset \mathscr{I}_{2,k^{(r)}} \right\}.$$

For $E^{(r)}$ such that $E^{(r)} \subset \mathscr{I}_{2,k^{(r)}}$, let us define the hypothesis that $p_i^{(r)} = p_1^{(r)}$ for $i \in E^{(r)}$ by $H^{(r)}(E^{(r)})$. Then

$$\bigwedge_{i \in E^{(r)}} H_i^{(r)} = H^{(r)}(E^{(r)})$$

holds.

Take the specific null hypothesis $H_{i_0}^{(r)} \in \mathscr{H}_2^{(r)}$. Then the closed testing procedure is to reject $H_{i_0}^{(r)}$ if the test of the null hypothesis $H^{(r)}(E^{(r)})$ is rejected at level α for any $E^{(r)}$ that satisfies $i_0 \in E^{(r)} \subset \mathscr{I}_{2,k^{(r)}}$.

We put $\ell := \ell(E^{(r)}) := \#(E^{(r)})$,

$$E^{(r)} := \{i_1, \cdots, i_\ell\} \quad (2 \leq i_1 < \cdots < i_\ell \leq k^{(r)}), \tag{9.14}$$

$$B_1(t|\ell+1, E^{(r)}) := \int_{-\infty}^{\infty} \prod_{j=1}^{\ell} \left\{ \Phi\left(\sqrt{\frac{\lambda_{i_j}^{(r)}}{\lambda_1^{(r)}}} \cdot x + \sqrt{\frac{\lambda_{i_j}^{(r)} + \lambda_1^{(r)}}{\lambda_1^{(r)}}} \cdot t \right) \right.$$
$$\left. - \Phi\left(\sqrt{\frac{\lambda_{i_j}^{(r)}}{\lambda_1^{(r)}}} \cdot x - \sqrt{\frac{\lambda_{i_j}^{(r)} + \lambda_1^{(r)}}{\lambda_1^{(r)}}} \cdot t \right) \right\} d\Phi(x),$$

$$\tag{9.15}$$

and

$$B_2(t|\ell+1, E^{(r)}) := \int_{-\infty}^{\infty} \prod_{j=1}^{\ell} \Phi\left(\sqrt{\frac{\lambda_{i_j}^{(r)}}{\lambda_1^{(r)}}} \cdot x + \sqrt{\frac{\lambda_{i_j}^{(r)} + \lambda_1^{(r)}}{\lambda_1^{(r)}}} \cdot t \right) d\Phi(x). \tag{9.16}$$

Furthermore, for a given α such that $0 < \alpha < 1$, we put

$b_1(\ell+1, \lambda_1^{(r)}, \lambda_{i_1}^{(r)}, \cdots, \lambda_{i_\ell}^{(r)}; \alpha)$
:= a solution of t satisfying the equation $B_1(t|\ell+1, E^{(r)}) = 1 - \alpha$, (9.17)
$b_2(\ell+1, \lambda_1^{(r)}, \lambda_{i_1}^{(r)}, \cdots, \lambda_{i_\ell}^{(r)}; \alpha)$
:= a solution of t satisfying the equation $B_2(t|\ell+1, E^{(r)}) = 1 - \alpha$. (9.18)

Then we have

$$\lim_{n \to \infty} P_{(r)0}\left(\max_{i \in E^{(r)}} |T_i^{(r)}| > b_1(\ell+1, \lambda_1^{(r)}, \lambda_{i_1}^{(r)}, \cdots, \lambda_{i_\ell}^{(r)}; \alpha) \right) = \alpha,$$

$$\lim_{n \to \infty} P_{(r)0}\left(\max_{i \in E^{(r)}} T_i^{(r)} > b_2(\ell+1, \lambda_1^{(r)}, \lambda_{i_1}^{(r)}, \cdots, \lambda_{i_\ell}^{(r)}; \alpha) \right) = \alpha.$$

[9.3] Multi-step Procedure for the Alternative Hypothesis of $H_i^{(r)A\pm}$

Take the specific null hypothesis $H_{i_0}^{(r)} \in \mathcal{H}_2^{(r)}$. If

$\max_{i \in E^{(r)}} |T_i^{(r)}| > b_1(\ell + 1, , \lambda_1^{(r)}, \lambda_{i_1}^{(r)}, \cdots, \lambda_{i_\ell}^{(r)}; \alpha)$ is satisfied, $H(E^{(r)})$ is rejected.
Then the closed testing procedure is to reject $H_{i_0}^{(r)}$ if the test of the null hypothesis
$H^{(r)}(E^{(r)})$ is rejected at level α for any $E^{(r)}$ that satisfies $i_0 \in E^{(r)} \subset \mathcal{I}_{2,k^{(r)}}$.

[9.4] Multi-step Procedure for the Alternative Hypothesis of $H_i^{(r)A+}$

Take the specific null hypothesis $H_{i_0}^{(r)} \in \mathcal{H}_2^{(r)}$. If

$\max_{i \in E^{(r)}} T_i^{(r)} > b_2(\ell + 1, , \lambda_1^{(r)}, \lambda_{i_1}^{(r)}, \cdots, \lambda_{i_\ell}^{(r)}; \alpha)$ is satisfied, $H(E^{(r)})$ is rejected.
Then the closed testing procedure is to reject $H_{i_0}^{(r)}$ if the test of the null hypothesis
$H^{(r)}(E^{(r)})$ is rejected at level α for any $E^{(r)}$ that satisfies $i_0 \in E^{(r)} \subset \mathcal{I}_{2,k^{(r)}}$.

9.3 Comparisons Under Order Restricted Proportions in the r-th Multi-sample Model

We assume that the simple order restrictions

$$p_1^{(r)} \le p_2^{(r)} \le \ldots \le p_{k^{(r)}}^{(r)} \tag{9.19}$$

are satisfied. The first treatment is regarded as a control with which the remaining
$k^{(r)} - 1$ treatments are to be compared. In one comparison, we test the null hypothesis
$H_i^{(r)} : p_i^{(r)} = p_1^{(r)}$ vs. the alternative hypothesis $H_i^{(r)A+} : p_i^{(r)} > p_1^{(r)}$. We put

$$\mathcal{H}_4^{(r)} = \{H_i^{(r)} \mid i \in \mathcal{I}_{2,k^{(r)}}\}. \tag{9.20}$$

Last, we introduce the procedure similar to the normal theory procedure of
Williams (1972). We assume the following condition:

(A7) $n_2^{(r)} = \ldots = n_{k^{(r)}}^{(r)}.$

Under the condition (A7), for ℓ such that $2 \le \ell \le k^{(r)}$, we define $T_\ell^{(r)}$ and $\hat{\mu}_\ell^{(r)}$ by

$$T_\ell^{(r)} = \frac{\hat{\mu}_\ell^{(r)} - \hat{v}_1^{(r)}}{\sqrt{\frac{1}{n_2^{(r)}} + \frac{1}{n_1^{(r)}}}} \text{ and } \hat{\mu}_\ell^{(r)} = \max_{2 \le s \le \ell} \frac{\sum_{i=s}^{\ell} \hat{v}_i^{(r)}}{\ell - s + 1},$$

respectively, where $\hat{v}_i^{(r)} := 2\arcsin\left(\sqrt{\hat{p}_i^{(r)}}\right)$.

Assume that $W_1^{(r)}, Z_2^{(r)}, \ldots, Z_{k^{(r)}}^{(r)}$ are independent and that $W_1^{(r)} \sim N(0, \lambda_2^{(r)}/\lambda_1^{(r)})$
and $Z_i^{(r)} \sim N(0, 1)$. We set

$$D_2^{(r)}(t|\ell, \lambda_2^{(r)}/\lambda_1^{(r)}) = P\left(\frac{\hat{\mu}_\ell^{(r)\Diamond} - W_1^{(r)}}{\sqrt{1 + \lambda_2^{(r)}/\lambda_1^{(r)}}} \le t \right), \qquad (9.21)$$

where $\hat{\mu}_\ell^{(r)\Diamond} = \max_{2 \le s \le \ell}\left\{\left(\sum_{i=s}^{\ell} Z_i^{(r)}\right)/(\ell - s + 1)\right\}$. Then under $H_0^{(r)}$,
$\lim_{n \to \infty} P_{(r)0}\left(T_\ell^{(r)} \le t\right) = D_2^{(r)}(t|\ell, \lambda_2^{(r)}/\lambda_1^{(r)})$ holds. We denote the solution of
$D_2^{(r)}(t) = 1 - \alpha$ by $d_2^{(r)}(\ell, \lambda_2^{(r)}/\lambda_1^{(r)}; \alpha)$, i.e., $D_2^{(r)}(d_2^{(r)}(\ell, \lambda_2^{(r)}/\lambda_1^{(r)}; \alpha)) = 1 - \alpha$.
When the assumption (A7) is satisfied, for $\alpha = 0.05,\ 0.025,\ 0.01$, the values of
$d_2^{(r)}(\ell, 1; \alpha)$ are stated in Tables 1 and 2 of Williams (1971). Shiraishi and Sugiura
(2015, 2018) give the algorithm based on sinc method to calculate $d_2^{(r)}(\ell, 1; \alpha)$. The
sinc method is described in Lund and Bowers (1992) and Stenger (1993). The algorithm is more efficient than that of Williams (1971).

[9.5] The Williams-Type Procedure
Whenever $d_2^{(r)}(\ell, \lambda_2^{(r)}/\lambda_1^{(r)}; \alpha) < T_\ell^{(r)}$ holds for any integer ℓ such that $i \le \ell \le k^{(r)}$,
we reject the null hypothesis $H_i^{(r)}$.

We put $\mathscr{I}_\ell := \mathscr{I}_{1,\ell} = \{i \mid 1 \le i \le \ell\}$ $(\ell = 2, \ldots, k^{(r)})$. For $\ell = 2, \ldots, k$, we
define $(\hat{v}_1^{(r)*}(\mathscr{I}_\ell), \ldots, \hat{v}_\ell^{(r)*}(\mathscr{I}_\ell))$ by $(u_1, \ldots, u_\ell)$ which minimize $\sum_{i=1}^{\ell} \lambda_{ni}^{(r)}$
$\left(u_i - \hat{v}_i^{(r)}\right)^2$ under simple order restrictions $u_1 \le u_2 \le \ldots \le u_\ell$, i.e.,

$$\sum_{i=1}^{\ell} \lambda_{ni}^{(r)}\left(\hat{v}_i^{(r)*}(\mathscr{I}_\ell) - \hat{v}_i^{(r)}\right)^2 = \min_{u_1 \le \ldots \le u_\ell} \sum_{i=1}^{\ell} \lambda_{ni}^{(r)}\left(u_i - \hat{v}_i^{(r)}\right)^2,$$

where $\lambda_{ni}^{(r)} := n_i^{(r)}/n^{(r)}$ and $n^{(r)} := n_1^{(r)} + \ldots + n_{k^{(r)}}^{(r)}$. Let us put

$$\bar{\chi}_\ell^{2(r)}(\mathscr{I}_\ell) := \sum_{i=1}^{\ell} n_i^{(r)}\left(\hat{v}_i^{(r)*}(\mathscr{I}_\ell) - \sum_{i=1}^{\ell}\left(\frac{n_i^{(r)}}{n^{(r)}(\mathscr{I}_\ell)}\right)\hat{v}_i^{(r)}\right)^2 \qquad (\ell = 2, \ldots, k),$$

(9.22)

where $n^{(r)}(\mathscr{I}_\ell) := \sum_{i=1}^{\ell} n_i^{(r)}$. We define $\tilde{v}_1^{(r)*}(\mathscr{I}_\ell), \ldots, \tilde{v}_\ell^{(r)*}(\mathscr{I}_\ell)$ by

$$\sum_{i=1}^{\ell} \lambda_i^{(r)}\left(\tilde{v}_i^{(r)*}(\mathscr{I}_\ell) - Y_i^{(r)}\right)^2 = \min_{u_1 \le \ldots \le u_\ell} \sum_{i=1}^{\ell} \lambda_i^{(r)}\left(u_i - Y_i^{(r)}\right)^2,$$

where $Y_1^{(r)}, \ldots, Y_\ell^{(r)}$ are independent and, for $i = 1, \ldots, \ell$, $Y_i^{(r)} \sim N(0, 1/\lambda_i^{(r)})$.
$P(L, \ell; \lambda(\mathscr{I}_\ell))$ becomes the probability that $\tilde{v}_1^{(r)*}(\mathscr{I}_\ell), \ldots, \tilde{v}_\ell^{(r)*}(\mathscr{I}_\ell)$ takes exactly
L distinct values, where $\lambda^{(r)}(\mathscr{I}_\ell) = (\lambda_1^{(r)}, \ldots, \lambda_\ell^{(r)})$. From the discussion similar to
(6.4), we get, under (A4),

$$\lim_{n\to\infty} P_{(r)0}(\bar{\chi}_\ell^{2(r)}(\mathscr{I}_\ell) \geq t) = \sum_{L=2}^{\ell} P(L, \ell; \lambda^{(r)}(\mathscr{I}_\ell)) P\left(\chi_{L-1}^2 \geq t\right) \quad (t > 0). \ (9.23)$$

For a given α such that $0 < \alpha < 1$, we put

$$\bar{c}^2\left(\ell, \lambda^{(r)}(\mathscr{I}_\ell); \alpha\right) := \text{a solution of } t \text{ satisfying the equation}$$

$$\sum_{L=2}^{\ell} P(L, \ell; \lambda^{(r)}(\mathscr{I}_\ell)) P\left(\chi_{L-1}^2 \geq t\right) = \alpha.$$

Then, we propose a stepwise procedure.

[9.6] Stepwise $\bar{\chi}^{2(r)}$ Procedure
Whenever $\bar{c}^2\left(\ell, \lambda^{(r)}(\mathscr{I}_\ell); \alpha\right) < \bar{\chi}_\ell^{2(r)}(\mathscr{I}_\ell)$ holds for any integer ℓ such that $i \leq \ell \leq k^{(r)}$, we reject the null hypothesis $H_i^{(r)}$.

9.4   Serial Gatekeeping Procedures

Suppose that the families $\mathscr{H}_2^{(1)}, \ldots, \mathscr{H}_2^{(q)}$ of null hypotheses have the order (9.3) of priority. Furthermore, suppose that, for some r, simple order restrictions $p_1^{(r)} \leq p_2^{(r)} \leq \ldots \leq p_{k^{(r)}}^{(r)}$ hold. Let us put the two sets

$$O_{1q} := \{r \mid p_1^{(r)} \leq \min\{p_2^{(r)}, \ldots, p_{k^{(r)}}^{(r)}\} \text{ is satisfied and } 1 \leq r \leq q\}, \qquad (9.24)$$

$$O_{2q} := \{r \mid p_1^{(r)} \leq p_2^{(r)} \leq \ldots \leq p_{k^{(r)}}^{(r)} \text{ is satisfied and } 1 \leq r \leq q\}. \qquad (9.25)$$

Then $O_{1q} \supset O_{2q}$ holds. We propose multiple test procedures for comparisons of

$$\{\text{the null hypothesis } H_i^{(r)} \text{ vs. the alternative}$$
$$H_i^{(r)A\pm} \text{ or } H_i^{(r)A+} \mid i \in \mathscr{I}_{2,k^{(r)}}, \ 1 \leq r \leq q\}, \qquad (9.26)$$

where we choose $H_i^{(r)A\pm}$ as the alternative hypothesis for $r \in O_{1q}^c \cap \{1, \ldots, q\}$ and choose $H_i^{(r)A+}$ for $r \in O_{1q}$. In Sects. 9.2 and 9.3, we state multiple tests among $p_1^{(r)}, \ldots, p_{k^{(r)}}^{(r)}$ for fixed r. In this section, we discuss multiple tests among $p_1^{(r)}, \ldots, p_{k^{(r)}}^{(r)}$ for all r's. Corresponding to (A4), we add the assumption of

(A6) $$\lim_{n^{(r)}\to\infty} \frac{n_i^{(r)}}{n^{(r)}} = \lambda_i^{(r)} > 0, \quad (1 \leq i \leq k^{(r)}, \ 1 \leq r \leq q).$$

Since the serial gatekeeping procedures are closed testing procedures, we introduce closed testing procedures for $\bigcup_{r=1}^{q} \mathscr{H}_2^{(r)}$.

The closure of $\bigcup_{r=1}^{q} \mathscr{H}_2^{(r)}$ is given by

$$\overline{\bigcup_{r=1}^{q} \mathscr{H}_2^{(r)}} \equiv \left\{ \bigwedge_{g=1}^{h} \left(\bigwedge_{i \in E^{(r_g)}} H_i^{(r_g)} \right) \; \middle| \; \text{there exist integer } h \text{ and integers } r_1, \ldots, r_h \right.$$

$$\text{such that } 1 \le h \le q, \; 1 \le r_1 < \ldots < r_h \le q, \text{ and}$$

$$\left. \emptyset \subsetneqq E^{(r_g)} \subset \mathscr{I}_{2,k^{(r_g)}} \; (1 \le g \le h) \text{ hold} \right\}.$$

Then, we get

$$\bigwedge_{g=1}^{h} \left(\bigwedge_{i \in E^{(r_g)}} H_i^{(r_g)} \right) : \text{for any } g \text{ such that } 1 \le g \le h \text{ and for any } i \in E^{(r_g)},$$

$$p_i^{(r_g)} = p_1^{(r_g)} \text{ holds.}$$

For nonempty $E^{(r_g)}$ such that $E^{(r_g)} \subset \mathscr{I}_{2,k^{(r_g)}}$, let us define the hypothesis that $p_i^{(r_g)} = p_1^{(r_g)}$ for $i \in E^{(r_g)}$ by $H^{(r_g)}(E^{(r_g)})$. Then we get

$$\bigwedge_{i \in E^{(r_g)}} H_i^{(r_g)} = H^{(r_g)}(E^{(r_g)}), \tag{9.27}$$

and

$$\bigwedge_{g=1}^{h} \left(\bigwedge_{i \in E^{(r_g)}} H_i^{(r_g)} \right) = \bigwedge_{g=1}^{h} H^{(r_g)}(E^{(r_g)}), \tag{9.28}$$

where $1 \le r_1 < \ldots < r_h \le q$.

[9.7] Hybrid Serial Gatekeeping Procedures

For integer r such that $1 \le r \le q$, in ascending order, perform multiple comparison test of level α based on stepwise procedure [9.3], [9.4], or [9.6], where we choose [9.3] for $r \in O_{1q}^c \cap \{1, \ldots, q\}$, choose [9.4] for $r \in O_{1q} \cap O_{2q}^c$, and choose [9.6] for $r \in O_{2q}$. Then we reject null hypotheses in $\bigcup_{r=1}^{q} \mathscr{H}_2^{(r)}$ obeying the following (b1)–(b3).

(b1) When there is a null hypothesis in $\mathscr{H}_2^{(1)}$ that is not rejected by the stepwise procedure [9.3], [9.4], or [9.6], only the null hypothesis rejected in $\mathscr{H}_2^{(1)}$ is rejected as a multiple comparison test of level α.

(b2) When there exists an integer q_0 satisfying $q_0 < q$ that, for any r such that $1 \le r \le q_0$, all the null hypotheses in $\mathscr{H}_2^{(r)}$ are rejected by stepwise procedure [9.3], [9.4], or [9.6] and there is a null hypothesis in $\mathscr{H}_2^{(q_0+1)}$ that is not rejected, all the null hypotheses in $\bigcup_{r=1}^{q_0} \mathscr{H}_2^{(r)}$ are rejected as a multiple comparison test and only the null hypothesis rejected in $\mathscr{H}_2^{(q_0+1)}$ is rejected.

(b3) When, for any r satisfying $1 \leq r \leq q$, all the null hypotheses in $\mathscr{H}_2^{(r)}$ are rejected by stepwise procedure [9.3], [9.4], or [9.6], all the null hypotheses in $\bigcup_{r=1}^{q} \mathscr{H}_2^{(r)}$ are rejected as a multiple comparison test of level α.

Theorem 9.1 *Suppose that the assumption (A6) is satisfied. Then the test procedure [9.7] is an asymptotic multiple comparison test of level α.*

Proof It is enough to show that [9.7] is a closed testing procedure of level α.

The test of level α for $H^{(r_1)}(E^{(r_1)})$ is executed. Furthermore, when $h \geq 2$ in (9.28), the test of level 0 for $H^{(r_g)}(E^{(r_g)})$ is executed for any g such that $2 \leq g \leq h$. As these results, we are able to decide whether or not the hypothesis $\bigwedge_{g=1}^{h} \left(\bigwedge_{i \in E^{(r_g)}} H_i^{(r_g)} \right)$ is rejected. Let us refer to this method as B-procedure.

(1). The case of (b1)

Suppose that $H_{i_1}^{(1)}$ is rejected by using the procedure [9.7]. Then, from B-procedure, $r_1 = 1$ holds and all the null hypotheses (9.28) satisfying $i_1 \in E^{(1)}$ are rejected. Suppose that $H_{i_2}^{(1)}$ is not rejected by using the procedure [9.7]. Then, from B-procedure, $r_1 = 1$ holds and some null hypothesis (9.27) satisfying $i_2 \in E^{(1)}$ is not rejected. Let $H^{(1)}(E_0^{(1)})$ be the null hypothesis that is not rejected. Then, from B-procedure, $H_{(i_2)}^{(1)}$ is not rejected. From B-procedure, $H^{(1)}(E_0^{(1)}) \bigwedge \left(\bigwedge_{g=2}^{h} H^{(r_g)}(E^{(r_g)}) \right)$ is not rejected. Therefore, all the null hypotheses in $\bigcup_{r=2}^{q} \mathscr{H}_2^{(r)}$ are not rejected.

(2). The case of (b2)

Since any null hypothesis (9.28) satisfying $1 \leq r_1 \leq q_0$ is rejected, for any r such that $1 \leq r \leq q_0$, all the null hypotheses in $\mathscr{H}_2^{(r)}$ are rejected. Suppose that $H_{i_1}^{(q_0+1)}$ in $\mathscr{H}_2^{(q_0+1)}$ is rejected by using the procedure [9.7]. Then, from B-procedure, $r_1 = q_0 + 1$ holds and all the null hypotheses (9.28) satisfying $i_1 \in E^{(q_0+1)}$ are rejected. Suppose that $H_{i_2}^{(q_0+1)}$ in $\mathscr{H}_2^{(q_0+1)}$ is not rejected by using the procedure [9.7]. Then, from B-procedure, $r_1 = q_0 + 1$ holds and some null hypothesis (9.27) satisfying $i_2 \in E^{(q_0+1)}$ is not rejected. Let $H^{(q_0+1)}(E_0^{(q_0+1)})$ be the null hypothesis that is not rejected. Then, from B-procedure, $H_{i_2}^{(q_0+1)}$ is not rejected. From B-procedure, $H^{(q_0+1)}(E_0^{(q_0+1)}) \bigwedge \left(\bigwedge_{g=2}^{h} H^{(r_g)}(E^{(r_g)}) \right)$ $(q_0 + 1 < r_2)$ is not rejected. Therefore, all the null hypotheses in $\bigcup_{r=q_0+2}^{q} \mathscr{H}_2^{(r)}$ are not rejected.

(3) The case of (b3)

From B-procedure, it is self-evident that all the null hypotheses in $\left\{ H_i^{(r)} \mid i \in \mathscr{I}_{2,k^{(r)}}, \ 1 \leq r \leq q \right\}$ are rejected.

From (1)–(3), the closed testing procedure of level α for (9.26) based on the B-procedure is equivalent to the procedure [9.7]. $\qquad \square$

Even if we replace [9.3] and [9.4] with [9.1] and [9.2], respectively, in the hybrid serial gatekeeping procedures [9.7], Theorem 9.1 still holds. Furthermore, even if we replace [9.6] with [9.5] in the hybrid serial gatekeeping procedures [9.7], Theorem 9.1 still holds under the condition (A7) of equal sample sizes.

9.5 Application to Multivariate Multi-sample Models

Let $\{X_{ij} = (X_{ij}^{(1)}, \ldots, X_{ij}^{(q)})^T \mid j = 1, \ldots, n_i, \ i = 1, \ldots, k\}$ be a set of independent vector-valued random variables. Then $\left(X_{i1}^{(r)}, \ldots, X_{in_i}^{(r)}\right)$ is a random sample of size n_i from the i-th Bernoulli population with success probability $p_i^{(r)}$ ($i = 1, \ldots, k$, $r = 1, \ldots, q$). It is convenient to assign the number 1 to a success and the number 0 to a failure.

$$P(X_{ij}^{(r)} = 1) = p_i^{(r)} \quad \text{and} \quad P(X_{ij}^{(r)} = 0) = 1 - p_i^{(r)}$$

hold. $X_{i1}^{(r)}, \ldots, X_{in_i}^{(r)}$ are assumed to be independent. We need not assume that $X^{(1)}, \ldots, X^{(q)}$ are independent, where $X^{(r)} := \left(X_{11}^{(r)}, \ldots, X_{kn_k}^{(r)}\right)$. Furthermore, the model is limited to

$$k^{(r)} = k \ (r = 1, \ldots, q) \text{ and } n_i^{(r)} = n_i \ (i = 1, \ldots, k, \ r = 1, \ldots, q). \quad (9.29)$$

The notations of $\mathscr{I}_{2,k^{(r)}}$ and $n^{(r)}$ are simplified to

$$\mathscr{I}_{2,k^{(r)}} = \mathscr{I}_{2,k} = \{i \mid 2 \leq i \leq k\} \text{ and } n^{(r)} = n = \sum_{i=1}^{k} n_i.$$

In the q variate k-sample model, the gatekeeping procedures [9.7] give multiple comparison tests of level α for all-pairwise comparisons of

$$\Big\{ \text{the null hypothesis } H_i^{(r)} \text{ vs. the alternative}$$
$$H_i^{(r)A\pm} \text{ or } H_i^{(r)A+} \Big| i \in \mathscr{I}_{2,k^{(r)}}, \ 1 \leq r \leq q \Big\}$$

under the limits of (9.29).

References

Lund J, Bowers KL(1992) Sinc methods for quadrature and differential equations. Siam

Maurer W, Hothorn L, Lehmacher W (1995) Multiple comparisons in drug clinical trials and preclinical assays: a priori ordered hypotheses. In Biometrie in der ChemischPharmazeutischen Industrie 6:3–18

Shiraishi T, Sugiura H (2015) The upper $100\alpha^\star$th percentiles of the distributions used in multiple comparison procedures under a simple order restriction. J Japan Statistical Society. Japanese Issue 44:271–314 (in Japanese)

Shiraishi T, Sugiura H (2018) Theory of multiple comparison procedures and its computation. Kyoritsu-Shuppan Co., Ltd. (in Japanese)

Stenger F (1993) Numerical methods based on sinc and analytic function. Springer-Verlag

Westfall PH, Krishen A (2001) Optimally weighted, fixed sequence and gatekeeper multiple testing procedures. J Stat Plan Inference 99:25–41

Williams DA (1971) A test for differences between treatment means when several dose levels are compared with a zero dose control. Biometrics 27:103–117

Index

© The Author(s), under exclusive license to Springer Nature Singapore Pte Ltd. 2022
T. Shiraishi, *Multiple Comparisons for Bernoulli Data*,
JSS Research Series in Statistics,
https://doi.org/10.1007/978-981-19-2708-9

Printed in the United States
by Baker & Taylor Publisher Services